FACE & BODY
CUPPING

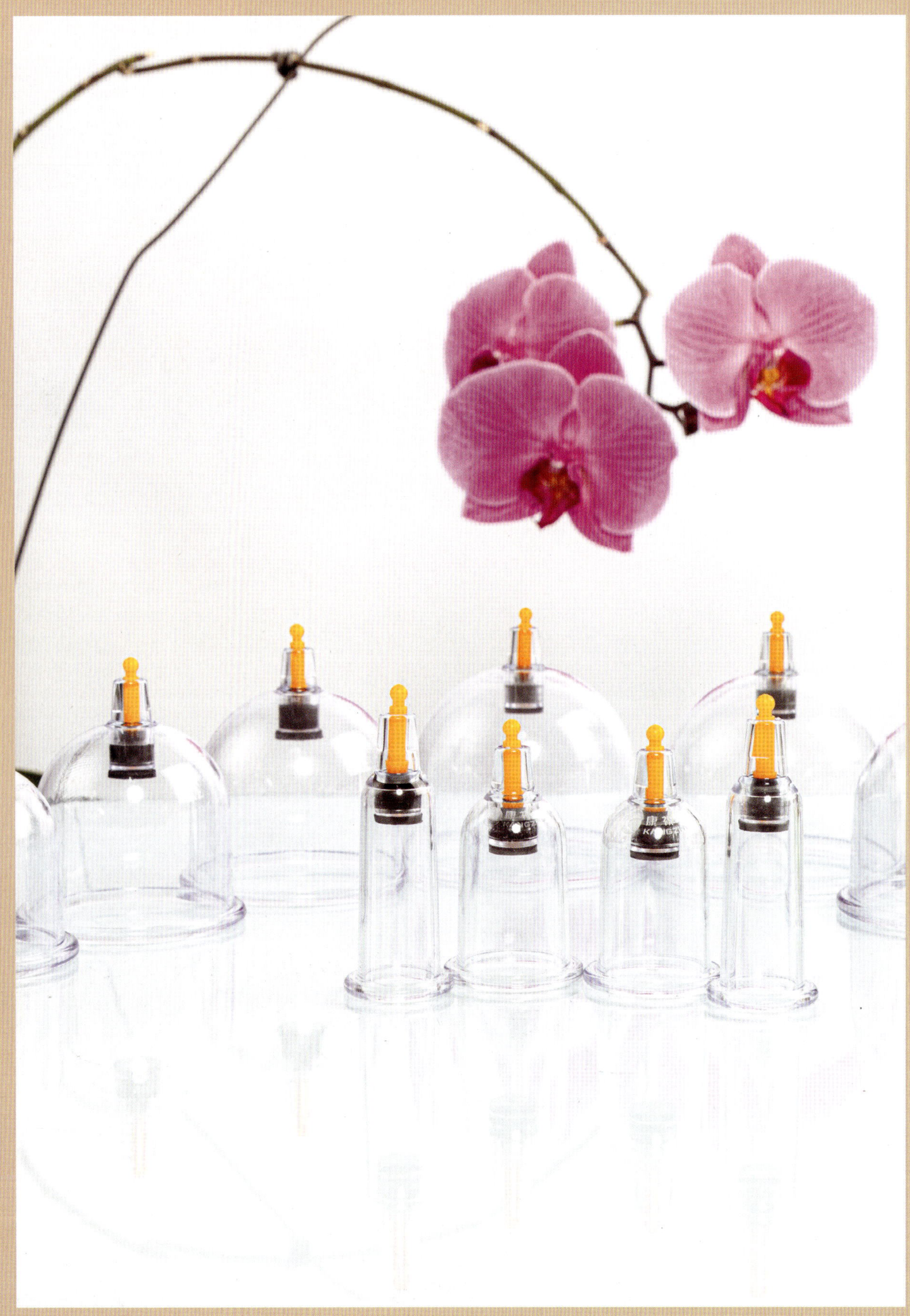

FACE & BODY CUPPING

A Step-by-Step Guide to Lymph Drainage for Professional Cosmetic Rejuvenation, Cellulite Reduction & Contouring

SHANNON GILMARTIN

CMT, CMLDT, CMCTPE

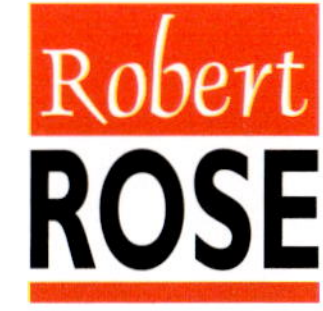

I dedicate this book to my family and
friends who have supported me on my
journey as a cupping educator and author.
And to all the professionals, clients and
cupping students who love the many
benefits of cupping bodywork.

CONTENTS

Part III: Body Cupping

INTRODUCTION

I love cups. With so many ways to use them, cups have become one of the most popular therapeutic tools employed and enjoyed by all types of bodyworkers. Whether they are being used by acupuncturists, massage therapists, physical therapists, athletic trainers or estheticians, cups can be incorporated into any type of hands-on treatment available today. When done correctly, they offer a whole new dimension of therapeutic benefit. From muscle relief and stress reduction to treatment of more complicated, pathological conditions, the healing effects of cupping are as diverse as its variety of applications. And with this wonderful range of therapeutic potential comes one of the most popular adaptations of cupping currently known the world over: cupping for cosmetic benefit.

In this book, you will find technical yet comprehensible explanations of how cupping affects the body on a physiological level. I examine the effects of cups, the physical responses they evoke and the relative anatomy involved with cupping for esthetic purposes, specifically the integumentary, circulatory and muscular systems. Additionally, in easy-to-follow, step-by-step detail, through text and in photos, I describe the two most popular treatments available using this style of therapeutic cupping: face cupping for cosmetic rejuvenation and body cupping for cellulite reduction.

This book will teach you how to offer safe and effective therapeutic cupping to reach the desired outcomes. Far too many people gain flawed information on the internet or from misinformed sources, and when they attempt these treatments, they do it incorrectly. Perhaps they leave cupping marks or bruises, cause pain or create swelling. Sadly, all of this is possible when cupping is done incorrectly. My goal with this book is to educate people on the best and safest methods to use in order to provide these treatments correctly and get the awesome results I know are possible.

I also discuss the different types of cupping equipment, using cups on the body, how to prepare the recipient for the best treatment possible and what to do afterward for maximum benefit.

And I address the million-dollar question: What about cupping marks? Neither of the cupping treatments covered in this book leaves cupping marks when done as instructed. In this book, you will understand exactly what a cupping mark is, why they occur, how to avoid the very small chance that cupping marks might appear, and what to do if they do.

This book also offers suggestions on how cupping can be tailored to fit everybody's personal needs, as no two people are alike. For the face, there are many opportunities to offer a variety of individualized detail. Is there loose skin to want to tone up? Cupping can help. Are wrinkles a primary concern? Cupping is a natural way to help reduce them. Does the overall complexion seem like it could use a little boost? Cupping can bring resilience back, naturally! For the body, you will learn how to focus on specific areas of cellulite concern, while also understanding how to address the entire body for optimal results. I've also included instructions and tips on how to enjoy both of these great treatments as self-care options.

Other personal needs are considered, too. For example, is there jaw tension related to TMJ dysfunction? Cupping can provide relief. Is there facial or body hair? There are recommendations on how to treat the entire body, whether there is hair or not. Is there acne? Sinus congestion? Have there been injections or other cosmetic procedures? Vascular considerations? More complicated, pathological concerns? If yes, there are suggestions on how to adjust the application so every person can enjoy the many benefits these applications of cupping have to offer.

As a professional bodyworker, cupping practitioner and international cupping instructor, I have had the opportunity to bring this great information to thousands of students and clients around the world. And for me, the journey into cupping bodywork all began after experiencing some truly remarkable effects first-hand. Every time I share my own history with cupping and the results, people either do not believe me, or they are shocked and even more excited to learn about these treatments for themselves. After years of chronic pain and scar tissue, cupping offered me extraordinary relief, and face cupping was transformational for me. If you want to read more about my personal story, turn to page 244 of this book.

After countless positive testimonials and amazing results, I look forward to sharing this information with you. I wish you all the success and fulfillment this type of cupping bodywork has to offer—enjoy!

This book offers suggestions on how cupping can be tailored to fit everybody's personal needs, as no two people are alike.

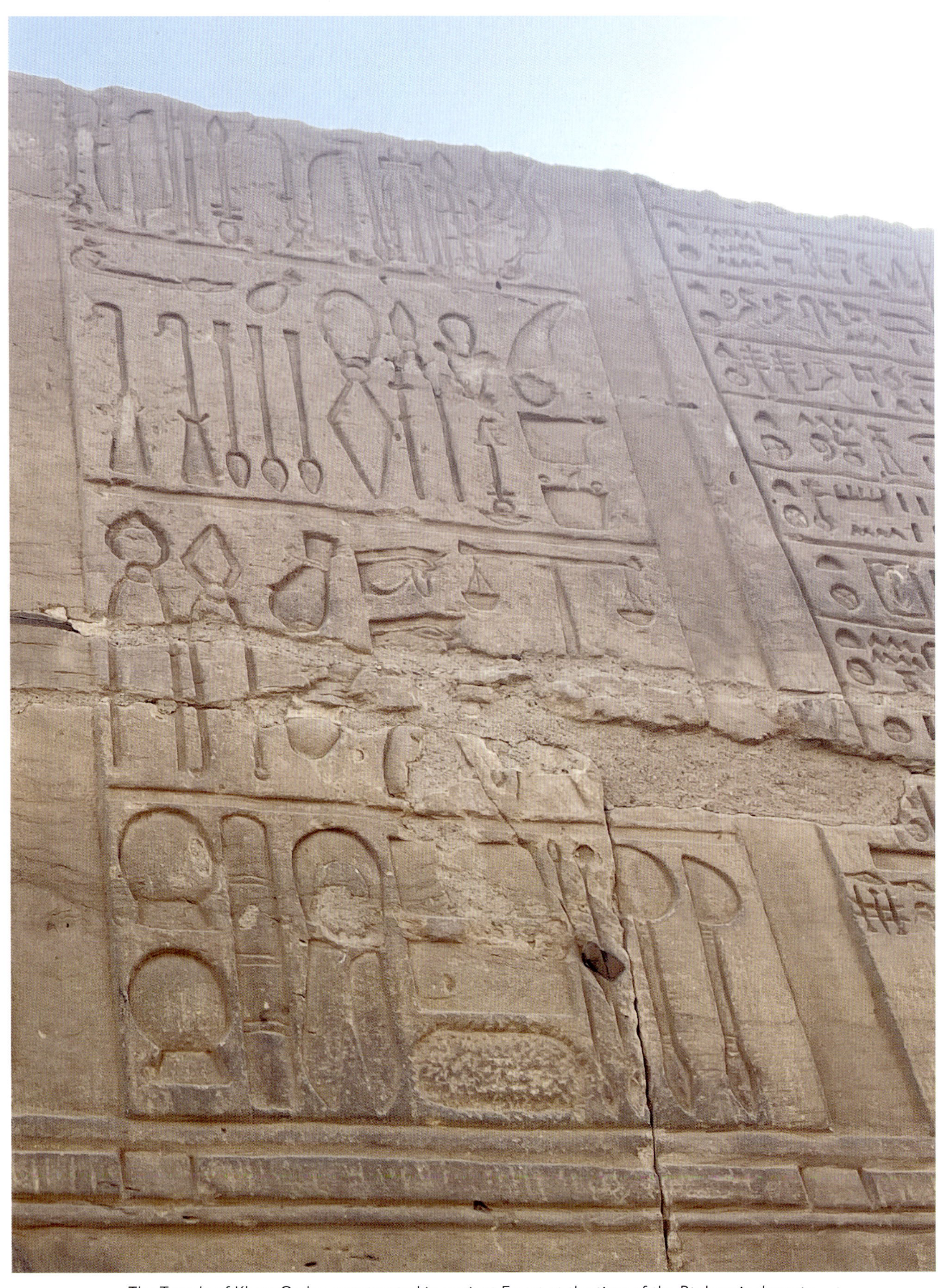

The Temple of Khom Ombo, constructed in ancient Egypt at the time of the Ptolemaic dynasty.
The stone carvings show medical instruments, including forceps, scalpels and (at the bottom left) cups.

History of Cupping

Cupping has been used throughout civilized times around the world. Its history goes back thousands of years to ancient Egypt, China, Greece, all over Europe and across the Americas. And while most records reference applications for a multitude of ailments—conditions such as musculoskeletal dysfunctions, pain relief, digestive issues, pulmonary afflictions, reproductive challenges, even expelling evil spirits—cupping for cosmetic purposes also has a rich history.

Cupping for cosmetic benefits can be similarly traced back to ancient Egypt, China, many European countries and even the Americas. In ancient times, only wealthy families and members of high society enjoyed the benefits of cupping for maintaining a healthy, youthful appearance.

More recently, in the twentieth century, when wellness spas began offering services for beauty, cupping devices began to be used along with various vibrational devices, scraping tools and other mechanical treatments. These early cupping treatments were used to reduce cellulite as well as other skincare treatments. More recently, in the 1970s and 1980s, there was growing interest in cupping for facial rejuvenation.

Nowadays, face cupping is one of the most popular noninvasive services available at premier wellness facilities. And while the clinical usages of body cupping have varied over the years, cupping for cosmetic rejuvenation has stayed strong in the wellness industry.

Although cupping is an alternative and complementary therapy used the world over, cupping results are difficult to measure by Western standards. As well, there are many interpretations of how to use them, and such confusion may result in inconsistent or improper usage. Cupping should never be painful. When done correctly, the results speak for themselves. People feel relief from cupping. You and your clients should find the experience of receiving cupping quite enjoyable!

With such a rich history, it is no wonder that today's cupping practices continue to provide relief and results unlike any other alternative manual therapy available.

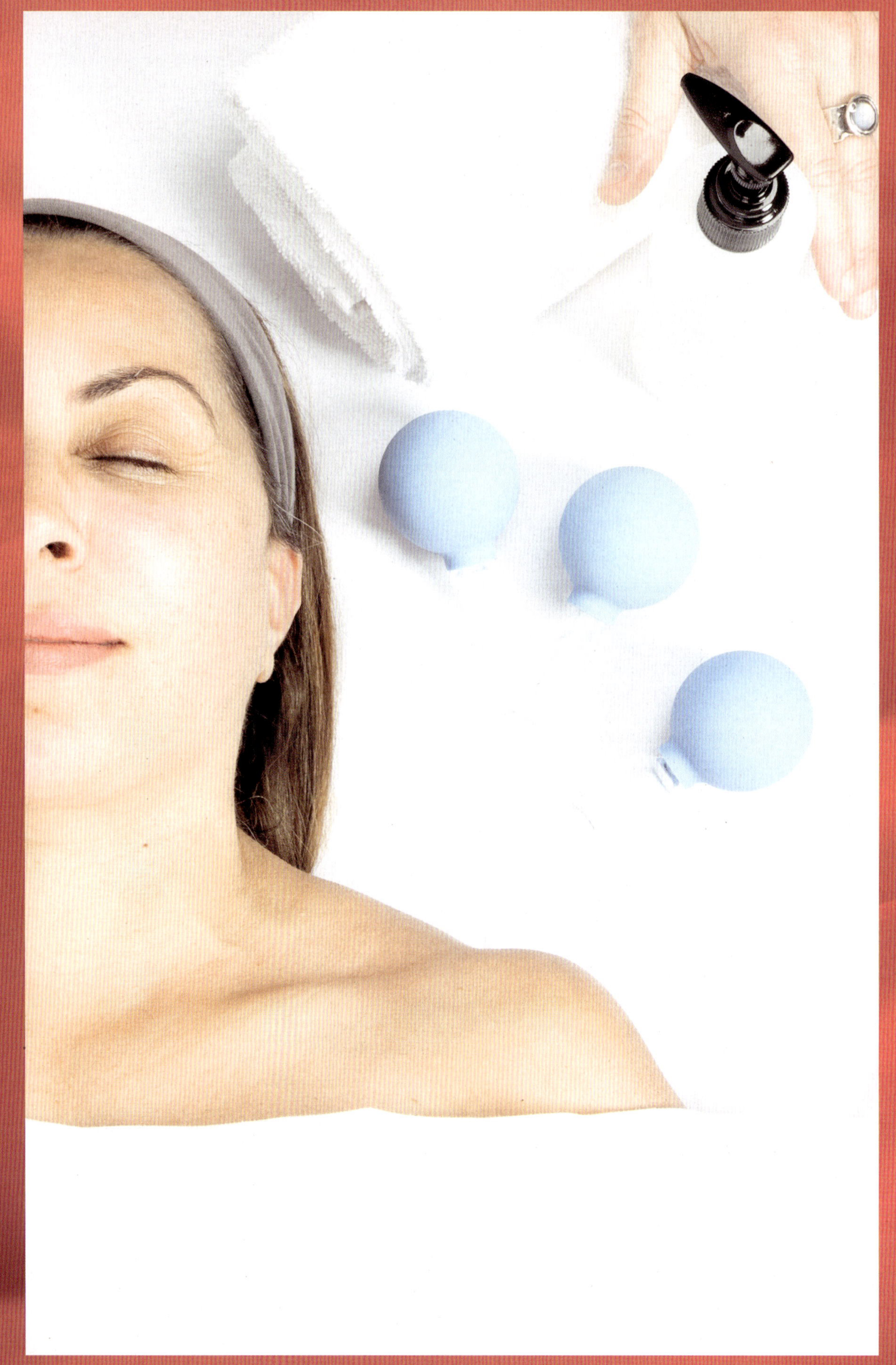

GETTING STARTED WITH CUPPING BODYWORK

CHAPTER 1

THE SCIENCE OF HOW CUPPING AFFECTS THE BODY

KNOW YOUR ANATOMY

This book is designed to inform the reader about cupping and its effects on human anatomy. To understand the contents, you will want to familiarize yourself with the following terms and anatomical details.

Body systems are the grouped organs and complementary body parts that make up our anatomy. Our body is made up of many systems, each with its own function. They include the integumentary, circulatory, muscular, skeletal, respiratory, digestive, reproductive, nervous, endocrine and exocrine systems.

The *circulatory system* is a body system that provides many vital functions and is broken into two subdivisions: the cardiovascular system, which controls blood movement, and the lymphatic (lymphovascular) system, which controls lymph movement.

Blood Vessels and Circulation

Blood circulates around the body through a complex network of vessels. Nutrient- and oxygen-rich blood leaves the heart via the aorta, which branches out into arteries that decrease in size to arterioles, eventually becoming minuscule capillaries.

At this microscopic level, blood is both distributed and begins its re-collection though a complex network of fluid-exchange processes known as *microcirculation.*

Venous return begins blood's route back to the heart. The venules (the smallest segment of veins) re-collect nutrient-deficient and deoxygenated blood from the capillaries, eventually becoming larger veins, which ultimately return to the heart via the superior and inferior vena cava. This deficient blood cycles through the right side of the heart, then travels into the lungs for oxygen replenishment before returning to the left side of the heart when the entire cycle begins again.

Capillaries are the smallest segments of bodily fluid moving vessels within the circulatory system. Blood vessels are involved with blood microcirculation, and lymph vessels are involved with lymph movement.

Lymph is a bodily fluid composed of cells (white blood cells, red blood cells, lymphocytes), proteins, water, fats (intestinal lymph), various metabolic waste products and other foreign substances. This fluid exists in the interstitial spaces of the body and is collected, filtered and circulated within the

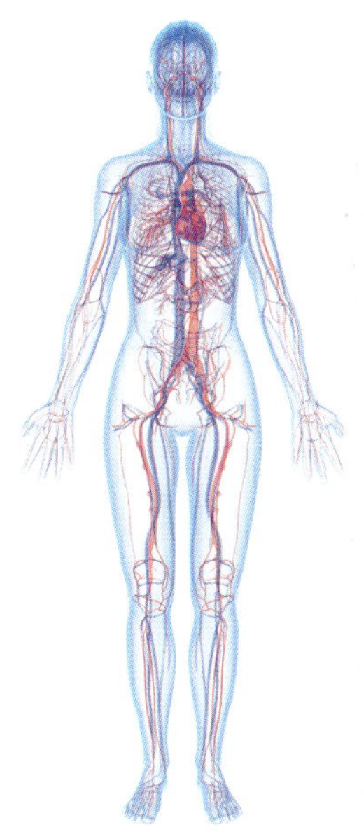

CIRCULATORY SYSTEM

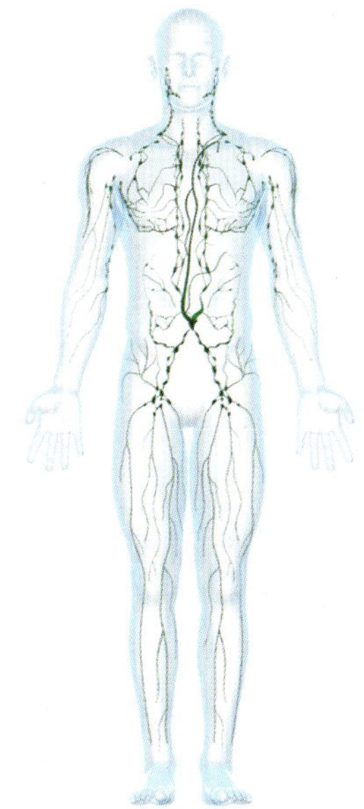

LYMPHATIC SYSTEM

many vessels of the lymphatic system. As a component of the circulatory system, lymphatic circulation is involved with maintaining bodily fluid levels of the body. Additionally, the lymphatic system serves important immunological functions.

Soft tissue is a general term used to describe various types of tissue structures in the body. While no tissue substance of the body is solid, bone is an example of a dense tissue structure. Soft tissue can be used to describe skin, muscle, fascia and even visceral organs. In this book, soft tissue is generally used to describe the more superficial layers of anatomy—skin, muscles and fascia.

Fascia is a form of connective tissue that exists in every part of the body. It is involved with every tissue structure (including skin, circulatory vessels, muscles, organs and bones), envelops every part of our anatomy and holds our bodies together.

Adhesions are defined as any two or more anatomical structures stuck together that shouldn't naturally be. These "stuck" areas are generally formed from injuries or inflammation but can also occur from a combination of repetitive muscle contractions, dehydration and poor circulation. Adhesions (also described as restrictions) can inhibit circulation, lymph drainage and muscle relaxation. This applies to face wrinkles that form between skin, muscle and fascia and also cellulite dimples that form over other locations on the body, such as the hips, thighs and abdomen.

PRIMARY PHYSIOLOGICAL RESPONSES TO CUPS ON THE BODY

Understanding how cups work on a physiological level provides some insight into why cups have been used for cosmetic enhancement and overall wellness throughout recorded history. While each body system will have a different reaction to cupping, there are a few basic physiological responses that occur when cups are applied to the body.

The primary physiological responses to cupping include:

- Negative pressure
- Vasodilation
- Enhanced fluid exchange

Keep these three physiological responses in mind as we progress into a deeper understanding of why cupping is so effective.

NEGATIVE PRESSURE

Once applied, cups lift the tissue and take effect with *negative pressure*. This is profoundly different from hands-on treatments such as massage therapy which use positive pressure, that is, pressing into the skin, to evoke a physiological response.

Ideally, soft tissues are hydrated, supple and pliable. However, there are many reasons that this healthy state of being can change, creating restrictions within the many layers of soft tissue. When soft tissues remain stuck together, adhesions form, contributing to soft tissue dysfunction on many levels.

One of the greatest positive effects of cups on the body is this negative pressure response within the layers of soft tissue, including skin, fascia and muscles. Rather than pressing, cups use negative pressure. This negative pressure creates a pulling action, which allows for the separation of fused or adhered tissue. Think of this negative pressure as plumping the skin, pulling in nutrient-rich blood flow and releasing indentations where tissues are compressed.

VASODILATION

Vasodilation is a physiological response to this applied negative pressure, which allows for blood and lymph vessels to expand, thereby improving their functions. When cups are applied, they stimulate a local response within the underlying tissue structures, promoting the release of vaso-activating chemicals such as acetylcholine, adenosine and histamines, which encourage blood vessels to dilate. This dilating response even affects the pores in our skin, aiding in cleansing the skin and helping it to better absorb skincare products.

Again, while hands-on treatments increase vascular dilation to encourage circulation of blood and lymph, cupping does this with negative pressure, which allows for the next response—enhanced fluid exchange—to be so powerful.

ENHANCED FLUID EXCHANGE

By activating vasodilation, cupping has a powerful effect on the movement of blood, lymph and interstitial fluids (fluids that surround cells). When capillaries are dilated, blood and lymph mobility are greatly enhanced. Cups act as a vacuum, drawing fluids into an area when applied. Then when they are removed, the processes of fluid uptake and recirculation are greatly improved, too. Cups boost blood distribution while also encouraging venous return and lymph fluid movement. This enhanced fluid-exchange combination of output and uptake has a wonderfully therapeutic, suction-pump effect on the body.

The combination of these three actions—negative pressure, vasodilation and enhanced fluid exchange—allows for some incredible reactions to take place within the body. This is especially true for the superficial layers of soft tissue that are involved with cupping applications for cosmetic purposes.

DID YOU KNOW?

People often report feeling itchy after cups have been applied. This is a common response to the increased histamines in the area caused by the vasodilating effects of the cups.

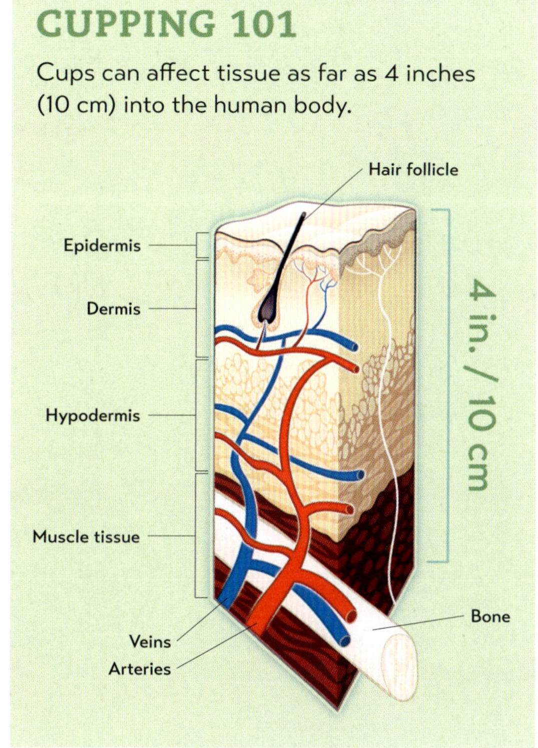

CUPPING 101

Cups can affect tissue as far as 4 inches (10 cm) into the human body.

THERAPEUTIC BENEFITS OF CUPPING

Through the combination of these primary physiological responses and various methods of application, there are many potential benefits to cupping bodywork.

- **Cupping encourages circulation.** One of cupping's most impressive benefits is that it stimulates overall circulation, even down to the capillary level, where it is known as microcirculation. Skin, muscles and even visceral organs all respond positively to the promotion of general circulation.
- **Cupping reduces adhesions.** Another benefit offered by cupping is that it addresses adhesions. The ability to lift and separate adhered tissue while also offering hydration to an area that was previously restricted is incredibly therapeutic. Adhesions can occur anywhere in the body, including the surface layers of the body, where they can appear as wrinkles or cellulite dimples.
- **Cupping helps clear congestion and stagnation.** Anything that is stagnant in an otherwise healthy internal environment can lead to a variety of illnesses and dysfunctions. Cups help clear stagnation from skin, muscles, bones, joints and organs. In some cupping practices, they are used to clear negative energies (whether emotional energies that lead to physical manifestations or energies relating to vital life forces, as with traditional Chinese medicine that uses cups to influence chi, or qi). Using cups for cosmetic purposes can clear out the internal stagnation of lymph fluids, blood or other waste materials that contributes to less-than-optimal esthetic appearances.

Cellulite

When cellulite forms, the dimpled adhesions that form between skin, muscles and fascia obstruct the general circulation of blood and lymph. The combination of adhesions and hindered circulation creates a vicious cycle of systemic stagnation and congested bodily fluids. Cups enable optimal fluidity and suppleness to return to the body by restoring circulation.

- **Cupping lifts, rehydrates and manipulates fascia.**
  Fascia is a form of connective tissue that can be smaller than a microscopic hair. It envelops all muscle tissues and is woven like a web throughout every part of the body, from inside the brain and blood vessels, to every organ and bone and the surface of the skin. It helps maintain the structural integrity of the entire body.

  Ground substance is a gel-like fluid that nourishes fascia, keeping soft tissues supple and pliable.

  Although fascia is flexible and yet durable, it can easily become restricted. Fascial restrictions contribute not only to cosmetic issues such as wrinkles and cellulite, but also more involved restrictions within the body, such as limited range of motion and other musculoskeletal dysfunctions.

  Fascial restrictions can be challenging to release with massage therapy or physical rehabilitation. Adding cupping to any of these therapies can help facilitate some impressive results. Cupping forces fluids to pass into and through the webbing of fascia. That can improve the hydration and pliability of what may be dehydrated and therefore adhered and restricted fascia. The negative pressure of lifting and stretching provides an opportunity to create suppleness where it is lacking. Cupping allows for some incredible therapeutic potential in otherwise challenged or immobilized areas.

- **Cupping can cause microtrauma in tissues.** Although this response sounds counterproductive, cupping can bring about microtraumas, or beneficial inflammatory reactions, when applied. When cups lift and pull soft tissues, these microtraumas occur in low-grade capillary and connective tissue levels, encouraging deep-seated restrictions to release. This rebuilds healthy tissue, thus encouraging the body's own process of healthy regeneration. This process allows for neovascularization to occur (see next item), which helps to stimulate collagen production while breaking up patterns of restriction like wrinkles or cellulite.

- **Cupping encourages neovascularization.**
  Neovascularization is the process by which new blood vessels form from existing healthy capillaries. Also known as angiogenesis, this microvascular regenerative process typically occurs in areas of injury or dysfunction (from cellulite dimples to scar tissue) where capillaries may be damaged or restricted.

PRESSURE CHECK: CUPS SHOULD NEVER BE PAINFUL

Although cupping causes beneficial microtraumas, cupping that is too strong can cause tissue damage. That is why it is so important to apply appropriate suction pressure. Cupping done in the manner described in this book typically uses a lighter suction pressure that will provide benefits. Regardless of the application, cupping should never be a painful experience.

When vasodilation and subsequent increased blood flow saturates the interstitial spaces surrounding the existing capillaries with a fresh supply of nutrients and oxygen, the result is a sprouting of new capillaries into the previously deficient soft tissues. This physiological response to cupping allows for a natural replenishment of vital nutrients such collagen and elastin, which contribute to the general health and overall appearance of skin.

- **Cupping helps alleviate excessive pressure on sensory organs in soft tissue.** This release leads to a reduction in pain. When soft tissue is restricted, it can cause the nerve endings that respond to various stimuli to become overactive, often resulting in a state of perpetual pain response. Cellulite or areas of wrinkles can be painful for some people when these nerve endings are "stuck" within these dimpled, adhered layers of soft tissue. The vasodilation response, along with the applied negative pressure, encourages these tight tissues to relax, thereby releasing the tension on the nerve endings involved. Unlike other cosmetic-focused therapies that rely on pressing into the body to get results and can be quite painful, cupping, in relying on negative pressure, can add pain relief to its cosmetic benefits.

- **Cupping reduces inflammation.** Inflammation is a natural process that occurs in the body for many reasons and on many levels. Every time a blood vessel dilates, it becomes inflamed. An inflammatory response is activated when an injury or sickness happens. Inflammation can also be a recurrent issue that affects the body on a systemic level and in a more pathological manner, with conditions such as rheumatoid arthritis and fibromyalgia.

  When inflammation occurs, the circulatory system produces an abundance of blood and lymph fluids to stabilize, heal and cleanse the inflamed area. The most notable symptoms of this response are localized swelling, palpable heat and pain at the site of inflammation.

When the inflammation dissipates, the body will slowly but surely remove the waste materials via lymphatic drainage. However, since lymph movement can easily become challenged—by example, from tight muscles or circulatory issues—massage or manual lymph drainage therapies are often recommended to clear restricted drainage pathways.

The influence on lymph movement is one of the most subtle yet powerful benefits of cupping when applied along drainage pathways. Adaptations of technique, methods of application and lighter pressure can have remarkable influence on the lymphatic system. The applications discussed in this book follow the lymph drainage pathways of the body.

Inflammation and Timing

Although cupping can reduce inflammation, it is contraindicated during times of acute inflammation, especially the initial 72 hours. Why? During those 72 hours, there is a surge of healing fluids and (if injury related) soft tissue reconstruction. If you drain the fluids away too soon, the body will produce even more of these fluids, which could cause excessive swelling. Further, the negative pressure pull of the cup could tear the tissues that are being mended. Cupping too soon would hinder the overall healing process.

If acute inflammation is in response to sickness, the person will feel sicker if cupped within 72 hours and may remain sick for longer since the cupping could circulate the sickness.

Still unsure? Ask your client to inquire with their health provider for medical consent to receive therapeutic bodywork before proceeding with cupping.

The exception here is for any certified manual lymph drainage therapists or health practitioners who have advanced training and knowledge of such conditions and appropriate treatment protocols.

BENEFITS FOR THE SKIN

The skin, which is part of the integumentary system, has many layers of soft tissue that contain nerves, hair follicles and glands, and hosts countless functions that all work together to regulate and protect the body. (The integumentary system includes the skin, hair, nails and some glands.) To understand healthy skin from the inside out, it is important to have knowledge of its anatomy and functions.

FUNCTIONS OF THE SKIN

- Skin protects the internal environment of the body from most external substances.
- It is a two-way, permeable barrier that both excretes and absorbs substances.
- Along with the circulatory and muscular systems, skin helps regulate body temperature and promote detoxification through perspiration.
- As an extension of the central nervous system, the skin is the first line of communication to the outside world, transmitting initial sensory input. Reactions to pressure, pain, temperature and environmental elements are first introduced to the body here.

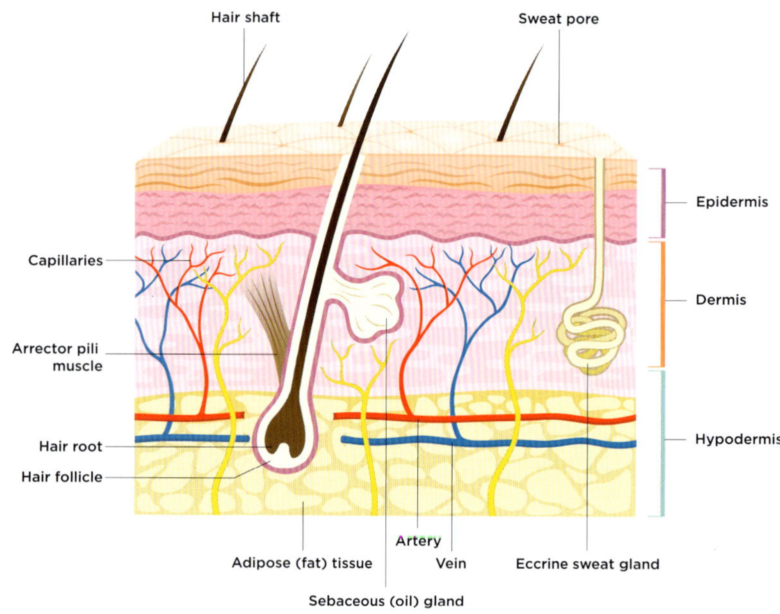

ANATOMY OF THE SKIN

Your skin has three primary layers: the epidermis, the dermis and the hypodermis.

The outermost layer is the *epidermis*. It is thin, offers protection and contains many nerve endings. It consists of epithelial tissues, which are avascular (lacking blood vessels) and therefore receive blood from underlying, connecting blood vessels by *diffusion* (see page 25). The epidermis is the last part of the body to receive blood flow, yet the first part we see, touch and feel.

The middle layer is the *dermis*, also known as the true skin. It supplies the skin with oxygen and nutrients thanks to its wealth of blood and lymph vessels. The dermis also contains collagen and elastin, which are protein substances that give the skin firmness and elasticity. As natural connective tissue cells called fibroblasts constantly work to rebuild tissues, they produce collagen and elastin; this is one of our normal cellular functions.

The deepest layer is the *hypodermis*. Also known as the subcutaneous or superficial fascia, this layer connects the skin to the underlying muscles. It is composed mostly of fatty (adipose) tissue, and contains many circulatory vessels, nerves and connective tissue fibers. Because this layer decreases with age, maintaining its wellness throughout our lives is vital to ensuring the health of the other, more superficial layers of skin.

NERVE ENDINGS IN THE SKIN

The dermis houses various *mechanoreceptors,* which are nerve endings, or sensory receptors, of the peripheral nervous system (see right). Whenever something touches the body, these receptors transmit this initial sense of contact along the peripheral nerves to the brain, where the brain processes this information and forms a response.

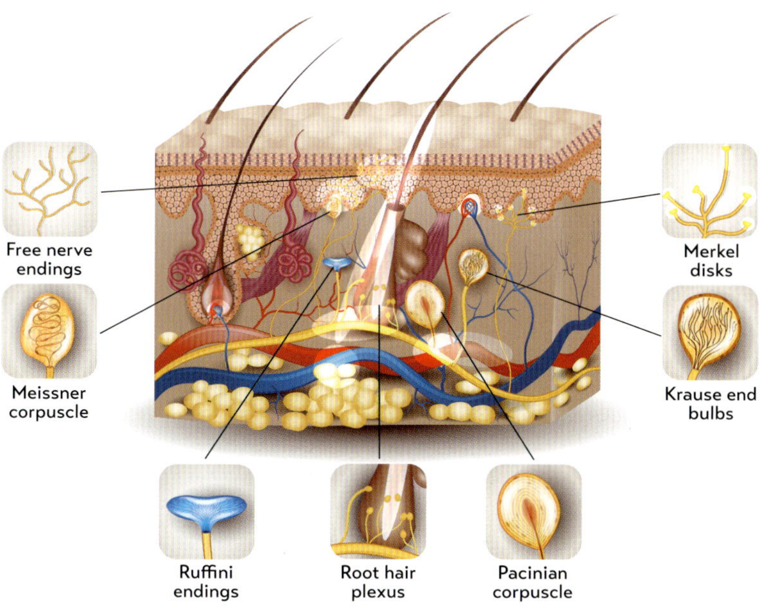

NERVE ENDINGS IN THE SKIN

ANATOMY FYI

Diffusion is the movement of substances from an area of higher concentration to one of lower concentration through a semipermeable barrier. For the skin, blood is diffused at the capillary level from inside the blood vessels out into the interstitial spaces to be absorbed and distributed to the surrounding soft tissues. **Interstitial** literally means the spaces within tissues.

ANATOMY FYI

COMMON SENSORY RECEPTORS

Nociceptors are nerve endings that respond to pain. They are located throughout the body especially in visceral organs, bone, joints, muscles and the skin.

Mechanoreceptors are located within the dermis and detect sensations such as pain, vibration and various applied pressures.

Thermoreceptors are located just under the surface of the skin within the dermis. They respond to temperatures both hot and cold.

Here's how sensory receptors work. Too much pressure from a massage can elicit one response (such as a "wincing" response within the muscles to tighten up and protect the body, or a verbal request to lighten up), while soft, soothing touch can bring about another (stimulating the parasympathetic nervous system, promoting circulation and relaxation).

The skin is the largest organ of the body and yet it is one of the last to receive blood nourishment. Maintaining a healthy appearance requires support not only from the outside but also, more importantly, from the inside body systems that nourish the skin. Although the composition of our skin is generally the same among all humans, individually our skin is what identifies us and gives each of us our own unique appearance.

Production of Collagen and Elastin in the Dermis

Our skin is nourished by blood, which contains many vital nutrients and organic substances that support its health. Among these substances are collagen and elastin, two primary nutrients necessary for maintaining a healthy, vibrant appearance. Mostly found in the dermis, both collagen and elastin are protein substances naturally produced throughout our lifetimes.

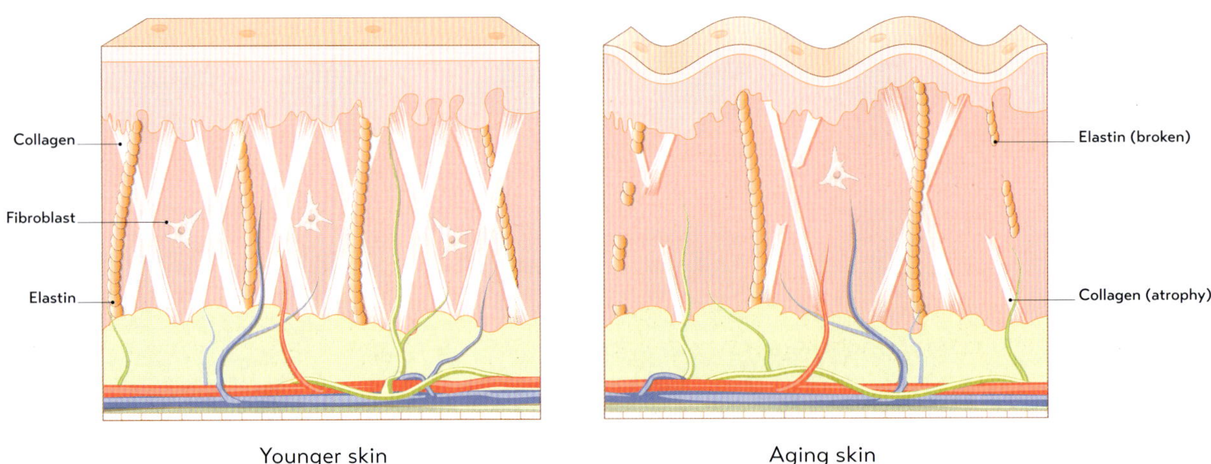

COLLAGEN AND ELASTIN PRODUCTION IN THE SKIN

Collagen makes up about 70 percent of the dermis; collagen fibers are protein-rich strands produced by fibroblasts, and are necessary for wound healing and general soft tissue construction. Elastin makes up much less in percentage—about 3% of the dermis consists of elastin fibers.

Both collagen and elastin give skin firmness and elasticity. As we age, natural production of these materials diminishes and skin loses elasticity. The resulting changes in appearance are something we all experience.

How Cups Improve Overall Appearance, Tone and Texture of the Skin

Since cupping boosts microcirculation, it provides detoxification and rejuvenation to all skin-covered surfaces wherever cups are applied. Add to that the low-grade microtraumas and the neovascularization that follows, and the production of collagen and elastin is stimulated. Adhesions involved with wrinkles and cellulite are lifted and softened, while the muscles involved are released and relaxed by the negative pressure.

As great as cupping is at reducing cellulite, it is important to acknowledge each client's response to pressure and sensitivity during the process. If cellulite is present, there can be existing discomfort if the nerve endings in the skin are already irritated from the restrictions associated with cellulite. It is easy to get overstimulated with some of the more vigorous, focused applications for cellulite focus areas. Simply put, a little cupping goes a long way. Be sure not to cause pain during any cupping treatments.

With all these elements combined, cupping brings about impressive benefits to the skin. We see skin tightening, a healthy glow surfacing and the general contours of the face and body becoming smoother and more defined.

BENEFITS FOR THE CIRCULATORY SYSTEM

Cupping has profound effects on the circulatory system. The skin is nourished, maintained and detoxified by the circulatory system, which exists throughout the many layers of the body. To understand the importance of blood and lymph circulation as it relates to cupping therapy, you need some knowledge of this complicated body system.

The circulatory system controls bodily fluids; in particular, it maintains blood and lymph circulation. For ease of understanding, we divide this complex body system into two parts: the *cardiovascular* and *lymphatic systems*.

The cardiovascular system is the part of the circulatory system that involves blood movement.

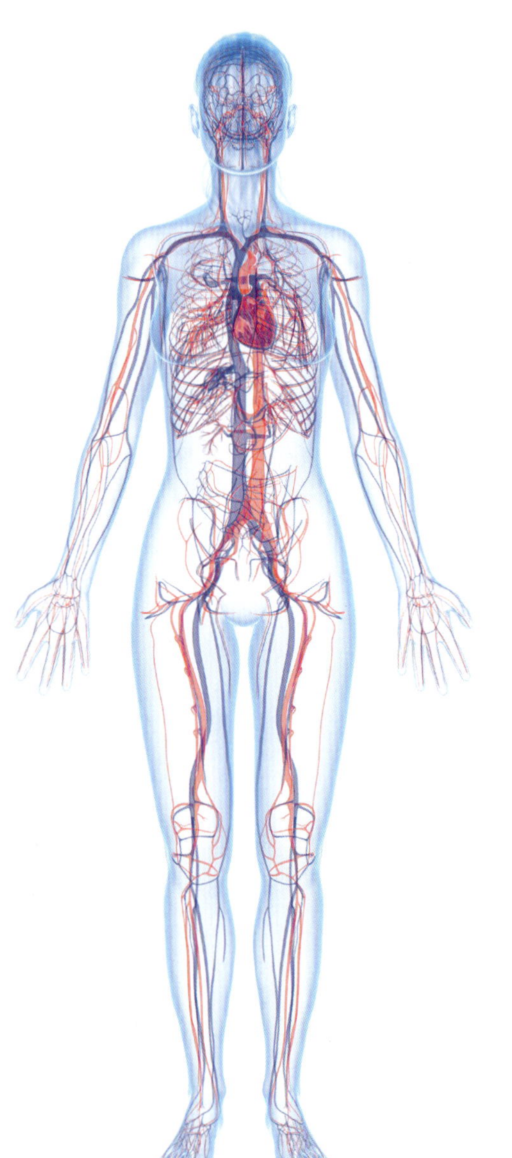

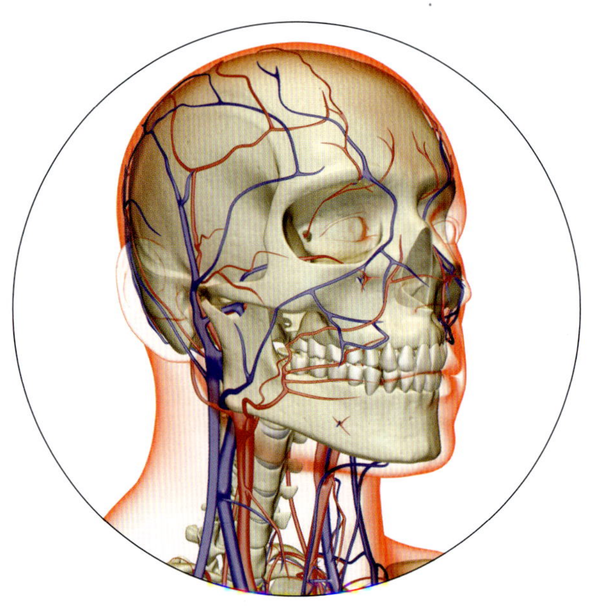

CIRCULATORY SYSTEM OF THE BODY (LEFT) AND THE HEAD (RIGHT)

FUNCTIONS OF THE CARDIOVASCULAR SYSTEM

- The cardiovascular system distributes respiratory gases (oxygen and carbon dioxide), nutrients, antibodies and hormones.
- It supports immune system functions by producing various disease-fighting cells, including red and white blood cells.
- It protects the body from excessive loss of bodily fluids from traumas by clotting.
- Along with the integumentary and muscular systems, the cardiovascular system helps regulate body temperature and promote detoxification through perspiration.

Blood vessels are tubes that carry blood both into and out of the heart, weaving throughout our bodies for thousands of miles. Blood distributes oxygen and vital nutrients—including those helping to produce collagen and elastin—into all parts of the body while simultaneously removing blood waste products. This distribution and waste removal exchange process, known as *microcirculation*, occurs at the capillary level.

Blood moves with various muscle contractions; when it leaves the heart, blood is pumped out through arteries, which decrease in size, eventually reaching the smallest segments, which are called capillaries. At these capillary end points are the venules (the smallest segments of veins) that collect nutrient-deficient blood and carbon dioxide waste. The venules progressively grow into larger veins—some identifiable under the skin's surface—ultimately ending at the heart where the cycle begins again.

At the skin level, we can easily identify a boost in blood circulation by a warming of the tissues and often also a pink coloring surfacing. This palpable and sometimes visible change is a response to increased activity within the dilated, inflamed capillaries.

Amid all this blood movement, blood also enters and exits the lungs, for carbon dioxide removal and oxygen replenishment. This cycle is constant and is vital to all of life's functions, especially overall health and wellness.

ANATOMY FYI

Arteries that distribute enriched blood are located deeper in the body than the veins that return deficient blood to the heart. Some of these veins are easily identified under the skin's surface, as in the temporal region around the eyes, the outer edges of the chest and the upper thigh region.

An Overview of the Lymphatic System

The other part of our circulatory system is the lymphovascular or lymphatic system, which controls lymph circulation. The lymphatic system exists alongside the cardiovascular system but has a circuitry all its own, involving many types of vessels, nodes and organs including the spleen, thymus gland and tonsils. Understanding the lymphatic system is equally important to promoting a healthy appearance and overall wellness, which is why we examine it here.

FUNCTIONS OF THE LYMPHATIC SYSTEM

- The lymphatic system maintains balance in the volume of bodily fluids.
- It filters lymph fluids and pathogenic substances, offering major defensive support to the immune system.
- It transports fats and vitamins from the digestive system into blood circulation.

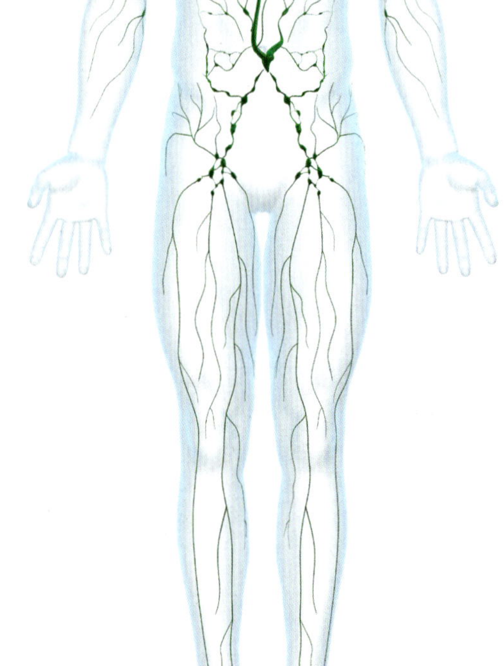

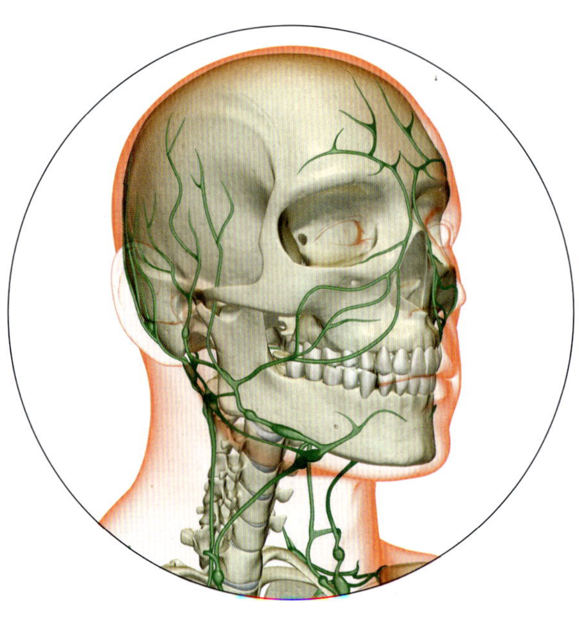

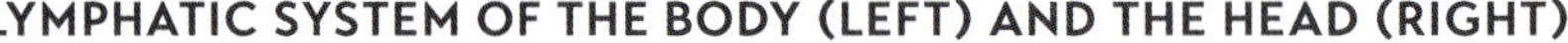

LYMPHATIC SYSTEM OF THE BODY (LEFT) AND THE HEAD (RIGHT)

WHAT IS LYMPH?

Lymph fluids consist of water, various cells, waste materials (including protein particles and metabolic waste not reabsorbed by the cardiovascular system during blood circulation) and any foreign or pathogenic substances such as environmental toxic exposures, bacteria and cancer cells.

The circulation of blood within the cardiovascular system controls the majority of the body's fluid-exchange processes. However, the small amount of fluid that escapes venous return at the capillary exchange remains in the space between tissues (interstitial of extracellular fluids), and this is where lymph is formed.

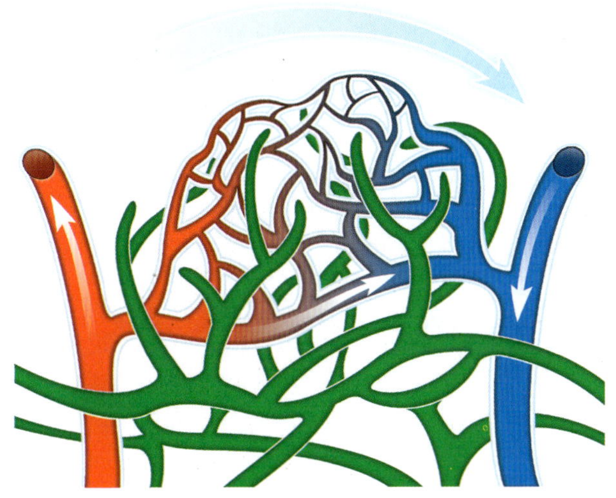

BLOOD AND LYMPH VESSELS

THE FLOW OF LYMPH

The lymphatic system follows its own complex drainage route, clearing lymph from sections of the body in a logical, holistic manner. Most of its collection begins at skin level with lymph capillaries, the "pre-collectors" that exist just under the skin and in the outermost layers of soft tissue. There are also lymph capillaries elsewhere in the body (such as within the digestive system) where additional lymph collection occurs.

Lymph capillaries are different from blood capillaries in that they contain specialized flap valves that respond to external pressure and open to allow lymph to enter the system. When an excess of interstitial fluid creates pressure on the flap valves, they open and try to accommodate as much of this fluid as possible.

LYMPHATIC SYSTEM 101

The lymphatic system is incredibly complex and has been extensively researched. While this book highlights only the points related to cupping, much is available from a variety of training programs offered around the world, such as by Dr. Emil Vodder's school of manual lymph drainage (www.vodderschool.com) and Dr. Bruno Chikly's health institute (www.chiklyinstitute.com). There are many reputable resources available if you want to more details on the complexity of this body system and its therapeutic manipulations.

LYMPHATIC ANATOMY FYI

Watersheds are lines of separation within the lymphatic drainage system. These delineated areas divide regions of the body to drain into specific collection areas for filtration at different sites of lymph node clusters.

The **thoracic ducts** (right and left) are located under the clavicle (collarbones), and are the end points for all lymphatic drainage and fluid recirculation. This is where filtered lymph fluids reenter blood circulation, at the subclavian veins.

- The *right lymphatic (thoracic) duct* drains lymph from the right arm, right side of the head and right half of the torso into the right subclavian vein.

- The *left thoracic duct* drains lymph from the rest of the body not taken in by the right thoracic duct into the left subclavian vein.

For more information on the full-body drainage pathways, see pages 174–175 in *Chapter 10: Body Cupping for Cellulite Reduction and Contouring.*

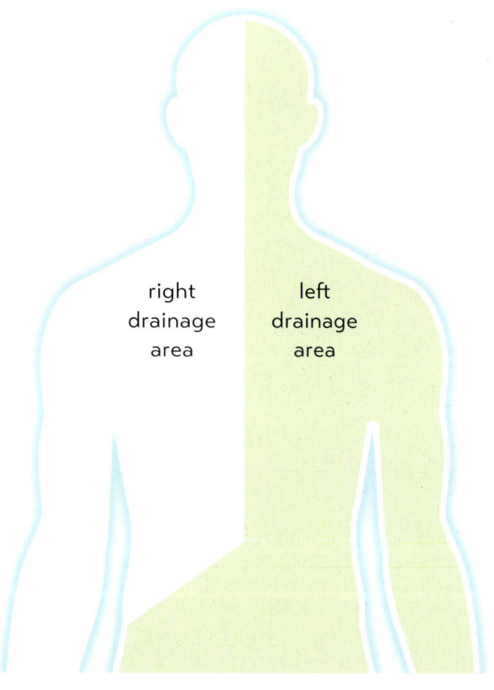

After collection, lymph fluids are moved along an intricate route of filtration and bodily waste removal. The entire body has a directional "map" of how lymph flows into the *thoracic ducts* (see *Lymphatic Anatomy FYI*, left).). Guiding this lymph flow, we have superficial collection regions located near the skin's surface, divided by *watersheds* (see left), that drain designated sections of the body. (See an illustration of the body's general flow of lymph drainage on page 175.)

From there, the lymphatic system progresses deeper into the body and further toward the core of the body in the torso, following specific routes of drainage. The lymphatic structures become larger and more complex; from superficial lymph capillaries, they grow into lymph vessels that move fluid along. These lymph "collectors" have flap valves similar to those within veins that prevent any backflow.

The lymph vessels lead into lymph nodes where much of the lymph is filtered; the average person has approximately 600 to 700 nodes. The lymph that remains is fed into lymph trunks (larger, more complex lymph components), and eventually into the two main drainage ducts in the torso (the right and left thoracic ducts) before reentering the blood circulation via the subclavian veins.

LYMPHATIC CHALLENGES AND THERAPEUTIC INTERVENTION

The movement of lymph can become altered and inhibited for many reasons, from injuries and surgeries to medications and personal habits (such as sedentary lifestyles).

Lymph generally moves by three mechanisms: breathing, muscle contraction and manual therapy. While we can breathe and activate muscle contractions on our own, manual therapies are very useful to promote lymph drainage.

For this reason, there is a specific skillset some bodywork and skincare professionals are trained in known as manual lymph drainage, or MLD. Since the lymph capillaries are located just underneath the skin, the highly trained hands of an MLD therapist applying light pressure can easily influence lymph drainage. Since the flow of lymph is easily influenced at this superficial level, following the correct drainage pathways is crucial. Lymph drainage treatments are a major component of most skincare professional services, and optimal lymph drainage is one of the best natural ways to improve and maintain healthy, beautiful skin.

The Importance of Blood and Lymph Circulation

If lymph fluids remain uncollected and stagnant, the interstitial spaces expand, thereby creating stagnation. If the lymphatic system becomes sluggish and overloaded, swelling occurs and the entire lymphatic system goes out of balance trying to remedy this excessive fluid congestion. If the volume of this fluid exceeds maximum capacity, the system cannot take it all in. This causes a sort of systemic backup that can escalate into even more serious issues, for example, edema, which is a swelling caused by too much fluid trapped in the body's tissues. Maintaining good lymph circulation is a continuous, systemic effort vital to maintaining the balance of bodily fluids.

If lymph intake and drainage is challenged, this creates a backup within the entire circulatory system. When this occurs, blood distribution is challenged since there is no interstitial "space" for blood to be distributed. Without blood distribution, nutrients and oxygen cannot reach their end points, including the skin's surface. Without both systems working at optimal output and intake, this backup causes skin to become malnourished, causing an overall unhealthy appearance and diminished function.

How Cups Stimulate Overall Circulation for Improved Esthetic Appearance

The world over, cupping therapy is favored for its influence on the circulatory system. Countless cosmetic treatments strive to improve circulation, but since cupping does this naturally, it is one of the easiest ways to achieve these benefits. Often a noticeable warmth and pinkness appears in the skin as blood circulation is boosted, indicating an immediate glowing response to cupping on the circulatory system.

With improved blood circulation comes a greater distribution of oxygen and stimulation of collagen and elastin production, which yields visible, palpable results for cosmetic benefit. And with such a dramatic increase of microcirculation comes an improvement in the collection of waste materials—the greater the output of healthy blood, the stronger the return of waste becomes.

The lymphatic system's response to cupping is equally profound. Because much of cupping activity happens at the skin level, gentle cupping has a powerful influence on both the uptake of lymph as well as its movement along drainage pathways.

Some of the most effective skincare treatments involve stimulating lymph drainage. For that reason, the cupping treatments described in this book follow general lymph drainage pathways and methods of application. Also, improved lymph drainage boosts blood circulation, creating a wonderfully balanced system of give and take, which ultimately contributes to an overall healthy appearance, healthy from the inside out.

Moreover, the subtle yet powerful responses to cupping within the circulatory system provide benefits that are noticeable and lasting, yet without the discomforts associated with other more invasive skincare treatments aimed at producing similar results.

BENEFITS FOR THE MUSCLES

A healthy muscular system is another major factor contributing to a healthy outer beauty. To understand how this system is involved in maintaining a healthy appearance, we must have knowledge of its basic anatomy, its involvement with circulation and its connection to the skin.

FUNCTIONS OF THE MUSCULAR SYSTEM

- Muscles help us to maintain posture and stability and move our bodies.
- They support overall circulation of blood and lymph through muscle contractions.
- They control smooth muscle activities in our visceral organs (such as the lungs and heart).
- Along with the integumentary and circulatory systems, muscles regulate body temperature and promote detoxification through perspiration.

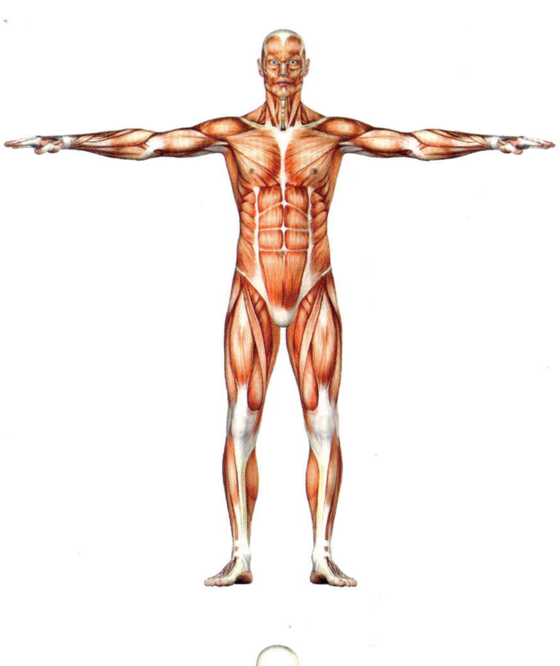

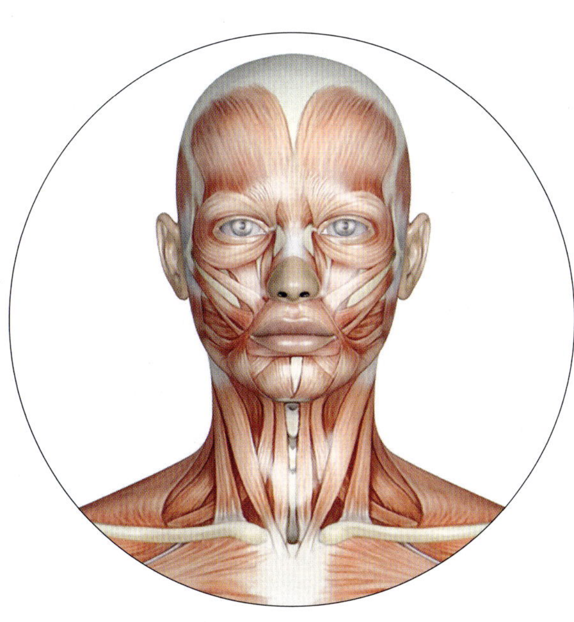

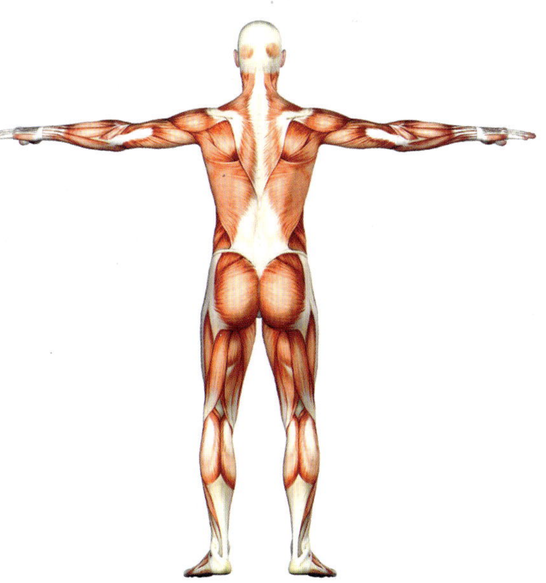

MUSCLES OF THE BODY

There are three types of muscles: skeletal, smooth and cardiac. The cardiac muscle is in the heart, and smooth muscles are predominantly in the visceral organs. Skeletal muscles are the ones responsible for movement, including facial expressions. Just under the skin are connections to the skeletal muscles and fascia.

Muscles contract and relax. With every action, blood and lymph is pumped along their circulatory routes with great efficiency. Muscle tissue also requires hydration to maintain suppleness and optimal function, from both daily water intake and from optimal internal circulation. Healthy muscle activity supports healthy circulation and healthy circulation supports healthy muscle function. Muscular adhesions, or restrictions, can affect layers of skin, muscle and fascia and can occur for many reasons.

Fascia is a type of connective tissue that is involved in every part of the body (see page 17 in *Know Your Anatomy*). These tissues exist throughout our anatomy in a continuous, web-like formation of collagenous fibers. Most connective tissue has a strong blood supply (is highly vascularized), and is nourished by its own fluid supply, including interstitial fluids and ground substance.

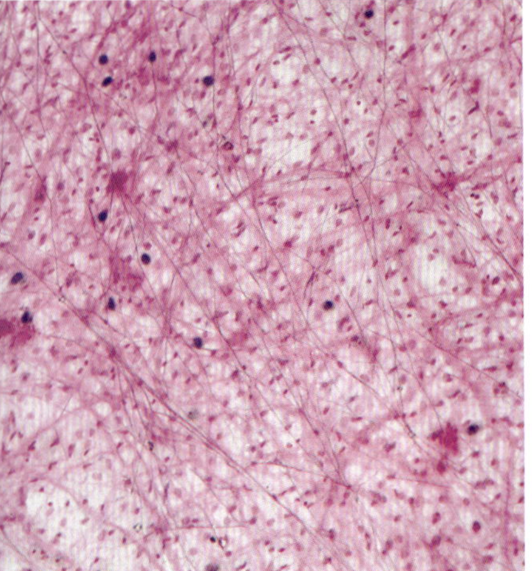

Fascia connective tissue fibers

FASCIA FACTS

Fascia is a subject of much research, especially in recent years. There are many websites, articles and books on the subject and its involvement with the human body beyond the material discussed in this book.

FUNCTIONS OF FASCIA

- Fascia supports and protects our body structure.
- It assists in the distribution of nutrients.
- It supports immune defense.
- It prevents blood loss (via clotting).

Fascia is responsible for the formation of blood, the dermis (inner layer of skin), superficial and deep fascia (fibrous tissue that keeps everything attached and connected), adipose tissue (stores energy and provides cushioning), bones, cartilage, ligaments, tendons and other thick, connective tissue structures such as aponeuroses. In summary, fascia is in every part of our bodies, especially the muscles.

Composed of collagen, fascia is very flexible and able to support bodily movements and adapt to physical stress and strain. If fascial pliability and ease of mobility becomes challenged, that can lead to restrictions, pain and other forms of physical dysfunction. Examples of fascial restrictions include cellulite, plantar fasciitis and frozen shoulder.

Understanding the Connection Between Muscles, Fascia, Wrinkles and Cellulite

To understand the connection between muscles, fascia and skin, we come back to adhesions. The bodily fluids that nourish fascia and muscle tissue flow into and through every aspect of this complex connective tissue system, helping all soft tissue structures to remain pliable and supple. Whenever this fluidity is challenged, adhesions can form. These restrictive adhesions inhibit circulation, lymph drainage and muscle activities. With these adhesions come a visible pulling of the outer skin surface. This inward pulling shows in the wrinkles that form in the face between skin, muscle and fascia, and in the cellulite dimples that form over other parts of the body.

How Cups Affect Muscles to Reduce Wrinkles and Cellulite

Cupping is such a great modality for addressing wrinkles and cellulite!

The negative pressure cupping provides gently decompresses all soft tissues—literally pulling on the wrinkles and cellulite dimples. This applied negative pressure encourages the circulation of blood into and through layers of muscle, improving not only muscle tone but also the systemic circulation of blood and lymph within the region. The negative pressure breaks up adhesive patterns that contribute to surface indentations, reestablishing smoother internal soft tissue anatomy with every treatment and, with time, its cumulative effects are incredibly therapeutic and lasting.

Cupping truly is one of the best noninvasive modalities for treating wrinkles and cellulite, and it works without discomfort or the adverse reactions associated with other treatments that claim similar results. We will further explore how cupping can be used effectively to reduce wrinkles in *Chapter 5: Face Cupping for Cosmetic Rejuvenation* and to tackle cellulite in *Chapter 9: Body Cupping for Cellulite Reduction and Contouring*.

MULTIFACETED BENEFITS

The goal of these treatments is to safely and effectively bring all the therapeutic benefits of cupping to the entire body, especially with the intention to improve overall soft tissue health and appearance.

Following the flow of lymph will simultaneously boost systemic circulation while smoothing muscle tension and relative adhesions.

This method of treatment reduces wrinkles, cellulite and discomforts associated with soft tissue dysfunction.

CHAPTER 2

CUPPING EQUIPMENT AND PRODUCTS

CUPPING EQUIPMENT

There are many types of equipment designed for various cupping applications. The most popular cupping sets are made of glass, silicone or plastic. There are also cupping machines that have become quite popular over the past few years, bringing cupping practices to a whole other level!

As with any product, it's important to work with the kinds of cups that best suit your personal or professional needs, preferences and budget. Some cups, such as silicone cups, are recommended for self-care treatments because they are easier to apply, while others, such as glass face cups, have benefits for the professional who is more comfortable working with such delicate items. Products vary in quality, functionality and durability, so purchase high-quality materials that work for you.

Of the many types of cups and cupping devices out there, the following are most recommended. They are simple to use, easy to clean and able to sustain the rigor of daily therapeutic bodywork. And while cups are sold in many places—health supply stores, pharmacies, bodywork educational companies, and even online—it is best to purchase units from a reputable source. (See *Resources*, page 248, for recommendations.)

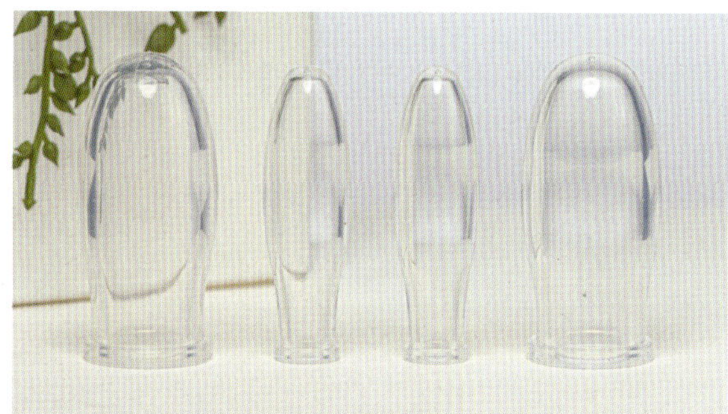

SILICONE FACE CUPS

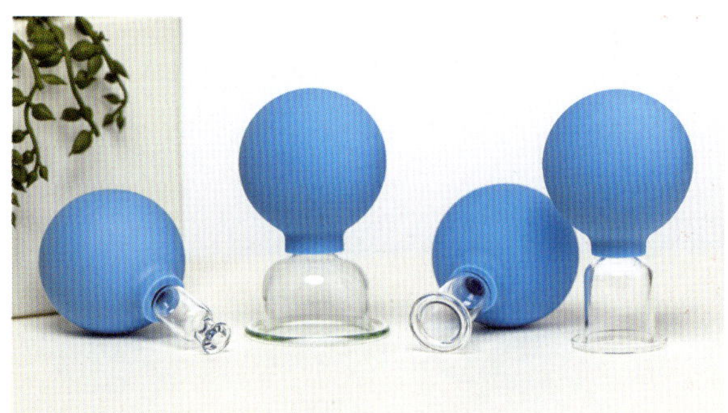

GLASS FACE CUPS

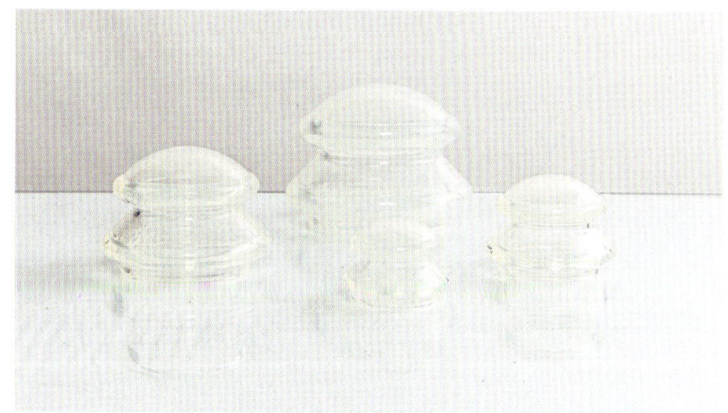

SILICONE BODY CUPS

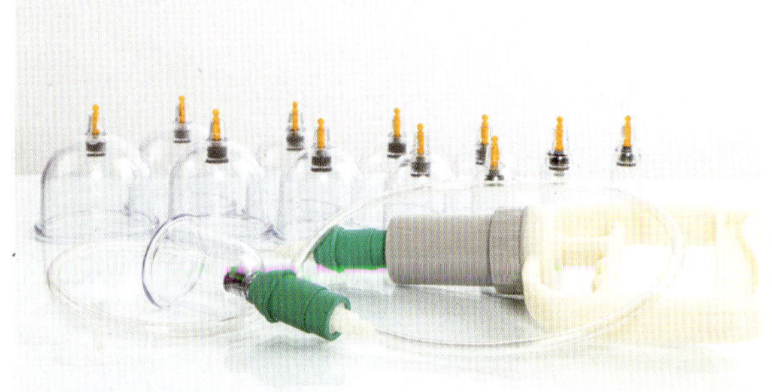

A MANUAL VACUUM PUMP CUPPING SET

Cupping Sets

FOR THE FACE

- **Silicone face cups.** These sets are good for personal and professional care and are usually sold with two or three cup sizes.
- **Glass face cups.** Due to their fragility and cleaning requirements, these are best for experienced practitioners.

Note: *For the purposes of this book, we focus on using glass cups for the face. Silicone cups are recommended for self-care use.*

FOR THE BODY

- **Manual pump cup set.** Featuring manual polycarbonate plastic cups with a vacuum hand pump, these sets are great for both professional and personal use. An easy-to-use hand pump creates the desired suction pressure. The wide variety of sizes run from large to very small to allow a full-body application for anyone interested in receiving cupping.

Note: *In this book, we focus on working with the manual pump cups for most of the body-cupping application and silicone cups for Cellulite Focus Options.*

- **Silicone cups.** These sets (with clear or slightly tinted cups) are good for personal and professional use but have a smaller range of sizes for full-body applications. Also, the constant need to squeeze the cups for proper suction pressure can be tiring for hands if used regularly in clinical practice.

Note: *For the applications in this book I recommend you use a manual pump cup set that has a detachable hose, used optionally to connect the hand pump to the cups.*

CUPPING MACHINES

There are some amazing cupping devices available on the market today, but they are intended for professional use only. Always be sure of proper operating functions, suction pressure and safety parameters when choosing to work with such electrical devices.

If you are a bodyworker looking for purchase options, see the *Resources* section on page 248 for contact information for high-quality cupping equipment distributors. You may also want to consider attending a live class to receive proper training on cupping machines.

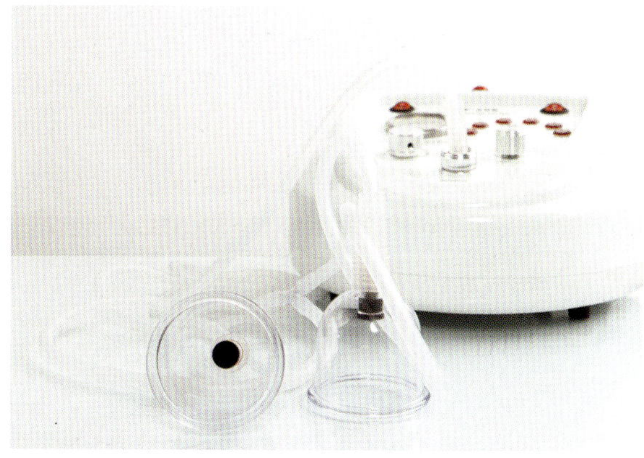

A CUPPING MACHINE

PRODUCT RECOMMENDATIONS

LUBRICANT

Before beginning any cupping bodywork, a lubricating medium must be applied to the skin. This is required for two reasons: to create a seal between the cup and the skin, and to make it possible to easily move a cup over the surfaces of the body.

The cupping applications described in this book require more "slip" across the skin than other traditional cupping practices. That makes a light, smooth oil the best option for these cupping treatments. For professional use, oils to consider include jojoba oil, fractionated coconut oil, fragrance-free sesame oil or almond oil.

For home care, there are many oils in your pantry that are great for your skin—I say if I can eat it, it can go on my skin! Some of the best options are olive oil or avocado oil, but any light, natural oil will do.

Some people may not want you to use oil on their skin, but using a quality oil is required for these treatments. Oil not only provides the necessary lubrication for cupping, but it also has hydrating, nourishing and protective properties for skin if you choose the right one.

CREAM OR LOTION

While oil is the recommended lubricant for these applications, any therapeutic quality cream or lotion can be of further assistance in a few instances.

These products work well on body hair and can be used in combination with oil (as needed) to create a good "slip" for the moving cups. Note that even when these products are used, cups may not adhere with excessive body hair.

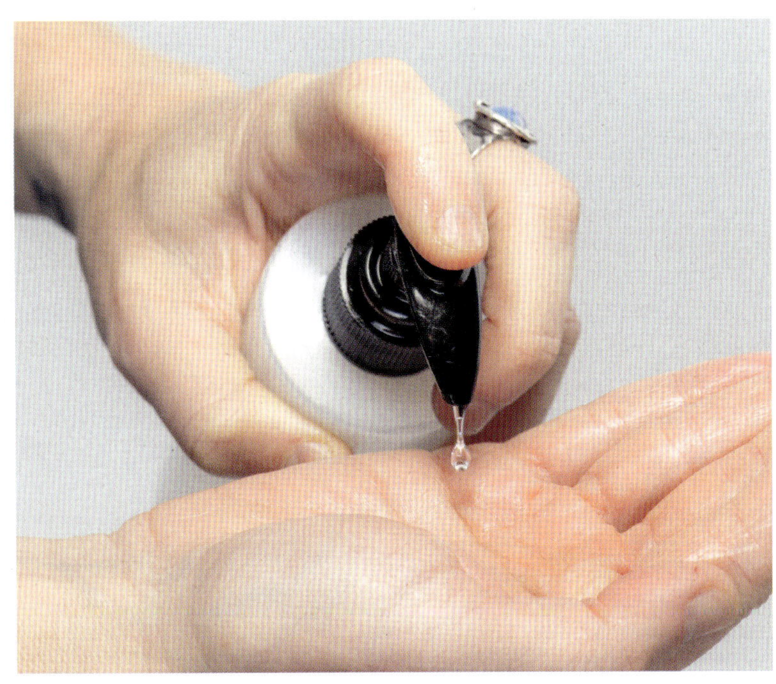

LUBRICATING PRODUCTS
Oil, cream or lotion are required for these cupping treatments.

Adding cream or lotion to oil may also help to create a smooth slide of the cup if skin is very dry.

Do not use lotion on the face, however, as it can clog pores. If you are working over facial hair, review the recommendations for Exceptions in *Chapter 6: Before You Begin Face Cupping.*

AMOUNT TO USE

No matter how much experience you have applying cups, this style of cupping requires a substantial amount of lubricant for best use, especially when attempting to slide the cups on the body. If there is too little lubricant, the cups will not move easily. That can be painful to the person receiving the work and may create cupping marks or bruises.

How much is required? You should use enough to create a thin layer on the surface of the skin but not so much that the oil is dripping off the body. For the face, the average face will require approximately a coin-shaped amount of oil. For the body, apply enough lubricant of choice so that the cup slides easily across whichever body part is being treated. The back will require more than the leg, and body hair or dry skin will be contributing factors to consider.

Apply plenty of oil at first, wipe it off your hands with a cloth or towel, then pick up the cups.

DO NOT USE

- **Do not use thick oils (for example grapeseed oil).** Thick oils are difficult to properly clean from the cup's surface and they don't have enough "slip" to move cups easily.
- **Do not use solid coconut oil.** While it is great for your skin care and absorption, it can congeal on the cup and be difficult to remove. Use fractionated coconut oil instead.
- **Do not use baby oil or mineral oil.** These types of oils are not recommended for skin treatments in general.

PROFESSIONAL TIP

Do not use expensive esthetics-grade face oil for the face cupping or costly cellulite oils for body cupping. I recommend using an oil that costs less since you will use a significant amount for each treatment, and that can become an expensive habit. Any high-quality face or cellulite oils would be great to apply after your treatment. See *Chapter 8: After a Face-Cupping Treatment* and *Chapter 11: After a Body-Cupping Treatment* for after-treatment recommendations.

CLEANING AND CARE OF EQUIPMENT

Cleaning

Washing your cups with antibacterial soap is the minimum requirement to ensure they have a long, clean life. Be sure to wash your cups in soap and water, then allow to air dry or wipe them dry if you need them sooner (for example, for your next appointment). While a simple washing is enough for self-care purposes, additional disinfecting of your cups is highly recommended and possibly required where you work. There are several products on the market that are approved for the silicone, plastic, or glass cups. (See the *Resources* section on page 248 for information on where to purchase them.)

If you encounter any blood or sebum—for example, if a pimple pops—you must disinfect your cups after they have been washed, whether for professional or personal use. For personal use, rubbing alcohol will work to disinfect the cup. For professional use, there are many great disinfectants that can be sprayed on the cups or wiped over their surfaces. There may be soaking processes required in some clinical settings also, so check the guidelines of your local health-care authority (the Centers for Disease Control and Prevention, local health department, etc.) to ensure proper cleaning standards are maintained.

Specialized Cleaning

MANUAL HAND PUMPS

Manual hand pumps should not be immersed in water. If water enters the pump, the internal mechanisms will corrode and break. The optional hoses should not be immersed in water either, as water in the tube can be drawn inside the hand pump as well. To clean, simply wipe them down with a slightly damp soapy cloth or approved cleaning wipes.

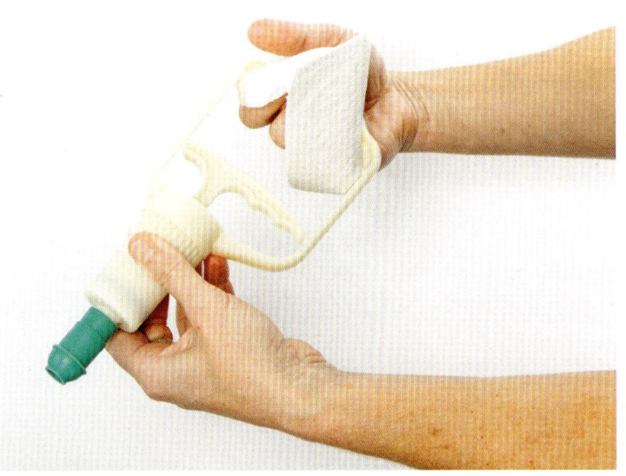

Do not immerse hand pump or hose in water; instead, wipe them down with approved cleansing and disinfecting wipes.

SQUEEZE BULB CUPS

Many glass face-cupping sets include squeeze bulbs to create the suction. Any squeeze bulb cups should be cleaned with caution. When washing the squeeze bulb, *be sure to wash only the outside of the bulb and do not get water inside the bulb.* Any water inside the bulb may cause mold to grow over time. If water does get inside the bulb, simply drip air dry, rinse the inside with alcohol and allow to drip air dry again. Try washing them with the opening of the bulb tipped down and out of the running water and be sure to also air dry with the opening tipped down.

The Limitations of Disinfecting Wipes

Disinfecting wipes do not fully clean the cups, and that can lead to cross-contamination when used in consecutive treatments. And over time, they will corrode and break down any non-glass cups. If using disinfecting wipes while working on-site (for example, at a house call or a sporting event), be sure to wash cups thoroughly in soap and water and disinfect them at the end of the day.

Storage

After they have been properly cleaned and dried, you may choose to store cups anywhere you prefer.

If working in your professional space, I recommend either storage racks or equipment carts that can both accommodate their storage and be cleaned as needed so they don't sit on dusty shelves.

For home use and self-care, you will want to put the cups away. You may choose to keep them in your medicine cabinet or wherever is convenient so you can readily access them for the next treatment.

Be sure not to store the cups with moisture in or on the cup, as mold may grow if the cups are left to retain moisture, especially when kept in dark spaces such as a cabinet or closet.

HOW TO USE CUPS

TECHNIQUES TO USE

HOW DOES CUPPING FEEL?

I have heard many different reactions to cups on the body. People say it feels stimulating and invigorating, soothing and relaxing. Some describe the sensation as a comforting lift and stretching of their skin and muscles, similar to what they feel with a great deep-tissue massage but without the pressure.

Every response will be unique and should be therapeutic. The one sensation a person experiencing cupping should not feel is pain. There are many ways to adjust cupping treatments to make it not painful—both with techniques and with pressure—so, if what you are doing results in any discomfort at all, stop. Adjust what you're doing as needed.

There are a variety of different techniques available when using cups. Many people, when they think of cupping, think of those bruise-like cupping marks—and we will discuss those marks later—however, the face- and body-cupping treatments described in this book are not those kinds of treatment. When it comes to using cups for face cupping or cosmetic body cupping, there are generally two techniques to use: lift-and-release and moving cups. I describe both techniques below as well as a combination of the two that most people use and which I call the Morse Code of Cups.

Treatment Photos

The treatment photos in this book have overlays to show the direction of movement and techniques to be used.

- The star marked on all cupping photos indicates the starting point(s).

- Where there are arrows (any line of movement), that means you can use lift-and-release or moving cups. The arrows point in the direction of the line(s) of movement.

- The Morse Code of Cups photo (on page 55) shows how lift-and-release and moving cups can be combined; this goes for any line of movement, anywhere on the body. Exceptions are the neck and delicate eye area, where only lift-and-release is used.

- A few cupping treatment photos (such as the Universal Pass on page 108) have only Xs marked on them. These indicate that this treatment process uses lift-and-release only.

- For the Cup-Free Options (as on page 77), the arrows show the direction in which your fingertips or hands will move.

Lift-and-Release

This is the most important technique to understand. It is an adaptation of both stationary (non-moving) *and* moving cups, intended to bring the benefits of cupping to the body without discomfort. You are literally "pumping" the tissue with a cup to facilitate quick changes in hydration, tension and pliability anywhere it's applied. Think of lift-and-release as milking the tissue into a healthier state.

In many clinical settings, cupping machines offer only this lift-and-release mode for face cupping because of how safe and effective it is. That is why this is the first technique to learn before moving on.

For face cupping, lift-and-release is used when you work down the neck, for every Universal Pass (see page 108) as well as in any tight or restricted areas (for many, that includes foreheads) where a moving cup simply doesn't move smoothly. For body cupping, it is used anywhere moving cups are not easily applied (as when moving over boney areas), or over hypersensitive or severely congested areas.

This technique is just as its name suggests. You lift the skin with a little suction for a moment and then simply release the suction and detach the cup from the skin. This gentle yet powerful technique lightly lifts skin and muscle and pumps the tissues, stimulating microcirculation and lymphatic activity. This technique is one of the best ways to introduce cupping to the body, as it takes effect without prolonged attachment.

TECHNIQUE FYI

For most of the treatments in this book, we don't use stationary cups; however, there is an option for a brief stationary cup over stubborn dimples in some of the Cellulite Focus Options.

Hard to Picture Lift-and-Release?

- To imagine the lift-and-release technique on the skin, visualize a jellyfish and the contraction (lift) and relaxation (release) of its body as it swims along.

- When manipulating the silicone squeeze cup, think of a duck's bill quacking; mimic this like a hand puppet with the cup in your hand to get used to the squeezing and releasing of the cup.

- The lift-and-release has plunger-like effects on the body—picture the movement of a plunger (slowly and gently, though) as you use it!

GLASS VERSUS SILICONE FACE CUPS

No matter what kind of face cups are used, the method of application is the same; silicone is squeezable and there are squeeze bulbs atop glass face cups.

HOW TO DO THE LIFT-AND-RELEASE TECHNIQUE

With silicone (squeeze) cups:

➤ Squeeze the cup, then lightly touch the cup to the skin's surface.

➤ Release the squeeze of the cup while maintaining your grip on the cup.

➤ Gently lift the cup away from the body until you feel a slight tension engage.

➤ Maintain the lift hold for approximately one second.

➤ Then release the lift and detach the cup from the skin; squeeze the cup again to release the suction.

➤ Do not yank the cup off—that will hurt.

With glass (squeeze bulb) cups, follow the same methods of application: squeeze the attached bulb to apply the cup, then squeeze it again to remove it.

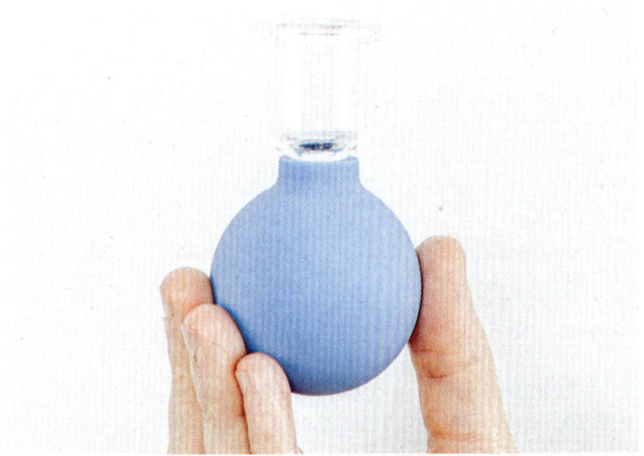
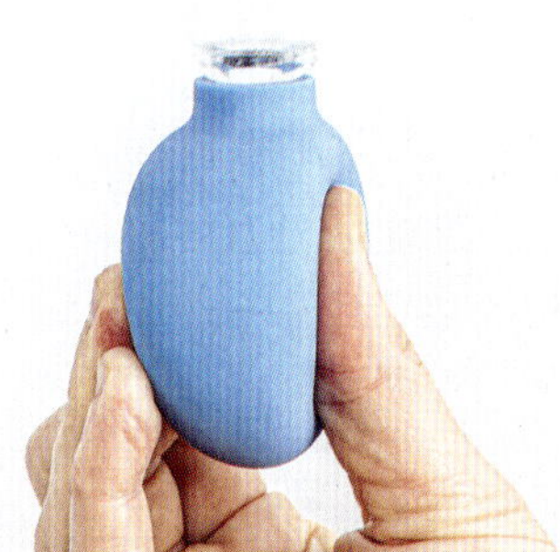

GLASS FACE CUPS WITH SQUEEZE BULBS

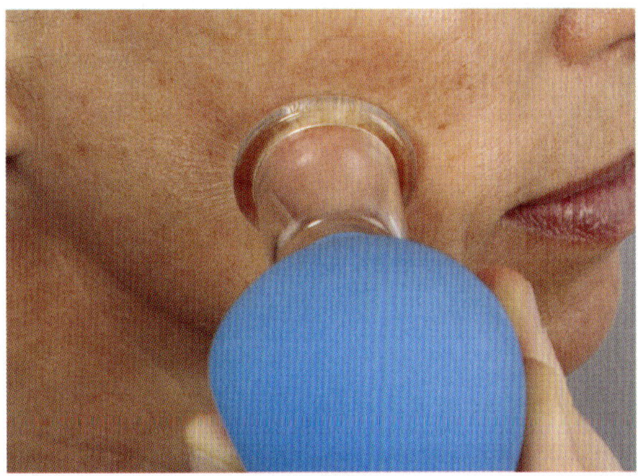

Correct lift-and-release with glass face cup:
Slightly lifting the cup away from the skin
while the cup is attached

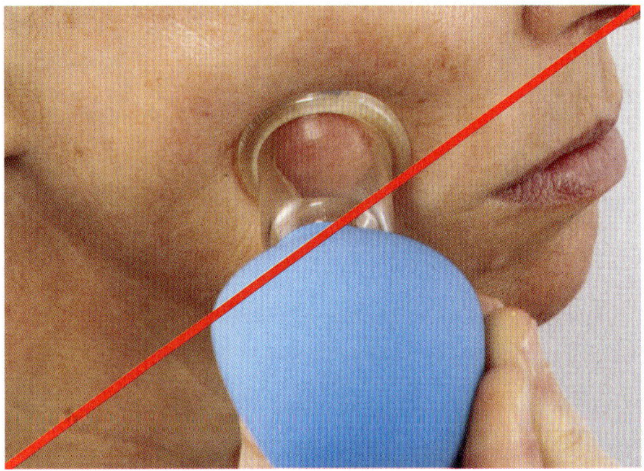

Incorrect:
Pressing the cup into the skin

With manual pump cups and the compatible hand pump:

➤ With manual pump in hand and cup attached (to the compatible hose), lightly touch the cup to skin's surface.

➤ Pump the trigger of the manual pump while maintaining your grip on the cup with your other hand.

➤ Gently lift the cup away from the body until you feel a slight tension engage.

➤ Maintain the lift hold for approximately one second.

➤ Then release the lift and detach the cup from the skin by sliding the pad of a fingertip under the outer edge of the cup, opening it away from you.

➤ Do not pop or yank the cup off without sliding your fingertip under the edge—that will hurt.

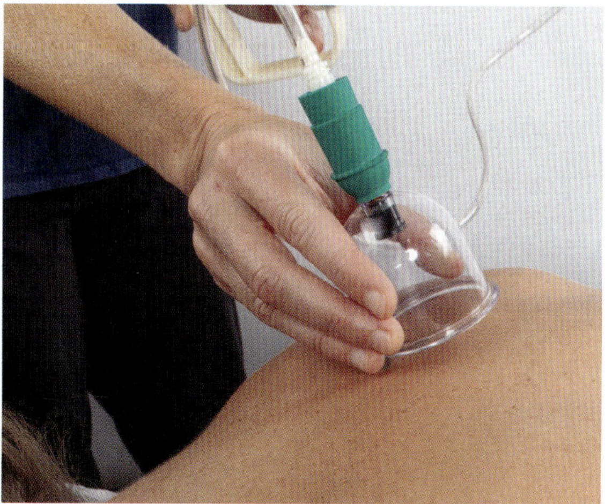

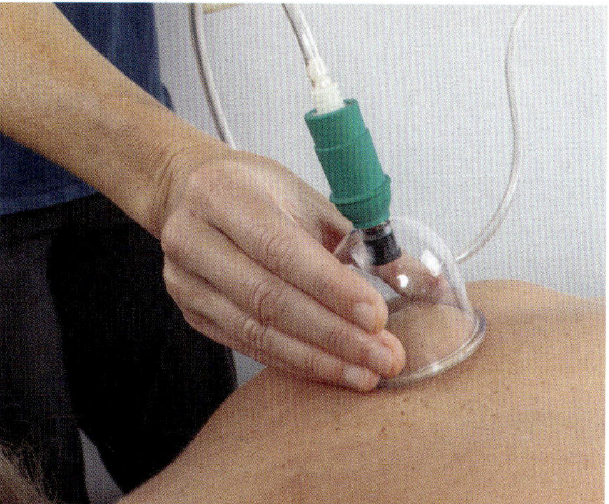

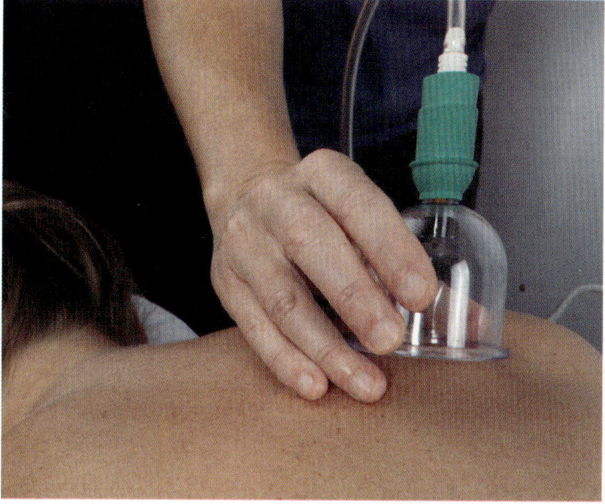

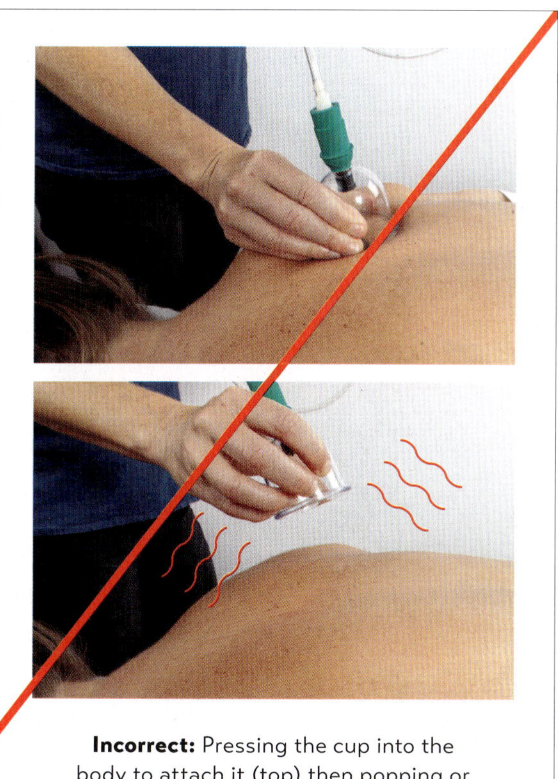

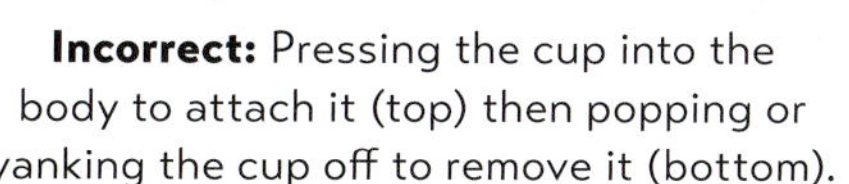

Incorrect: Pressing the cup into the body to attach it (top) then popping or yanking the cup off to remove it (bottom).

Correct lift-and-release with manual pump cup on the body: Attaching the manual pump cup with pump gun and compatible hose (top), creating suction with a "lift" to the cup (center), then releasing the cup from skin with the fingertips (bottom).

ATTACHING AND REMOVING SILICONE BODY CUPS

Silicone cups are recommended for Cellulite Focus Options.

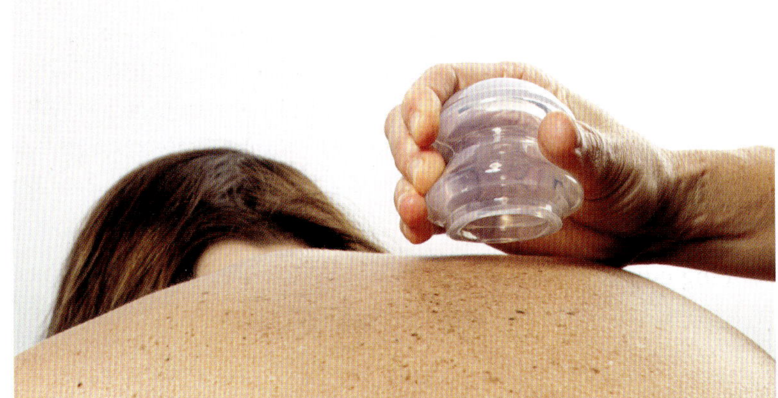

➤ First, squeeze the cup before making contact with the skin.

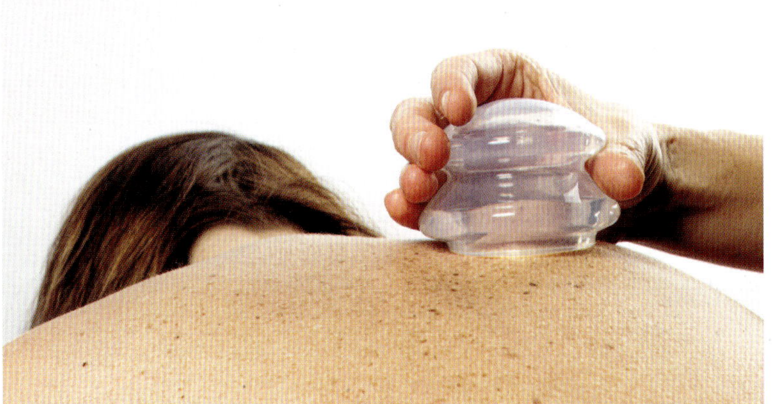

➤ Then, release the squeeze of the cup while maintaining the grip of it while you move it across the skin's surface.

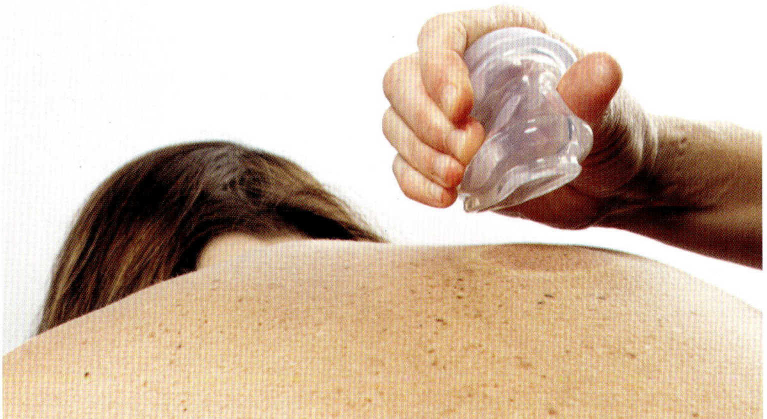

➤ When done using the cup, simply squeeze it again to detach it from the body.

Moving Cups

Moving cups feel wonderful when done correctly!

With every slide of the cup, your client will feel a softening, toning and overall revitalizing sensation. Imagine a vacuum cleaner (but a soothing, small and silent one) stimulating circulation, promoting the removal of lymphatic debris and smoothing out the surface layers of soft tissue everywhere it is moved.

Moving cups generally move more easily with repetitive, cumulative usage. This means that the more the internal fluid-exchange processes take place, the more hydrated and therefore more pliable the tissue becomes, making for an easier slide of the cup with every pass. Often, the first few passes over any area may be challenged because the applied lubricant is insufficient and/or there is a lack of soft tissue pliability. Lift-and-release will help to soften any "stuck" spots from the inside out, eventually allowing for easier moving cups thereafter.

Be sure to have ample lubricant applied and do your best to make it a smooth move.

HOW TO DO THE MOVING CUPS TECHNIQUE

➤ *These instructions apply to moving cups with any cupping set.*

➤ Attach the cup to the skin using lighter pressure.

➤ Gently lift the cup away from the body until you feel a slight tension engage.

➤ While maintaining this lifted hold, slowly begin to slide the cup across the surface of the skin.

➤ Then release the lifted tension and detach the cup from the skin, either by squeezing the cup again (if a squeeze cup) or with the pads of your pinky and/or ring finger fingertips (as described with manual pump cups).

➤ Do not yank the cup off—it will hurt.

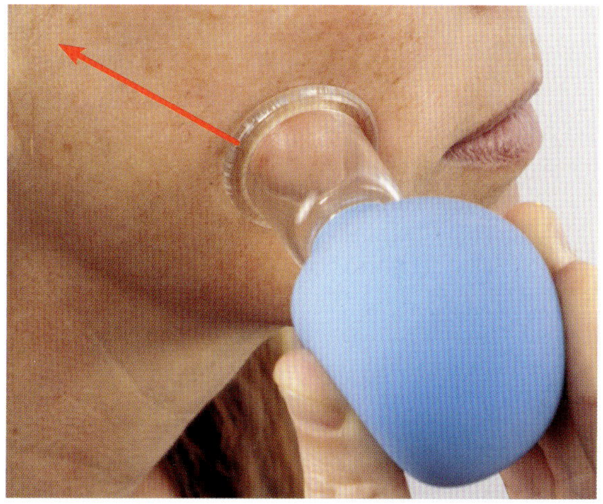

Correct moving cup with glass face cup:
Sliding the glass cup across the skin's surface while maintaining contact, slightly lifting the cup as you move it along

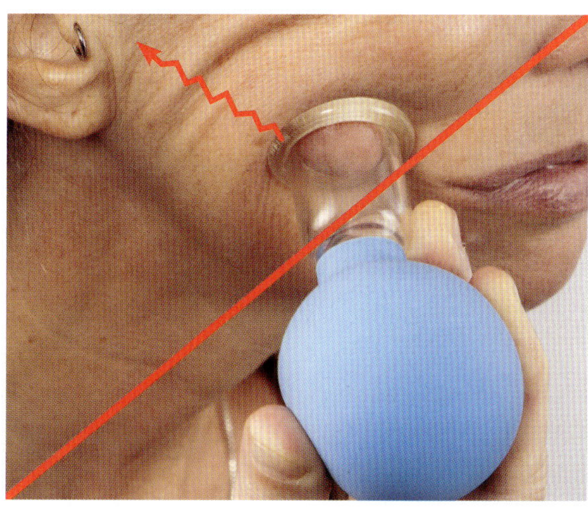

Incorrect moving cup with glass face cup:
pressing the cup into the skin, trying to drag it across the surface. If done incorrectly, you will notice a backup of skin in front of the cup and the cup may be difficult to move.

Benefits of Lifting a Cup on the Body

Why lift the cup as you use it? Adding a little lift of tension to any applied cup not only adds benefit to the layers of anatomy, but also makes it easier to move over the surface of the body.

For example, body cupping for cellulite and contouring is often done with too much suction pressure, resulting in pain, tissue damage and bruising. For better, safer results, use lighter suction pressure and lift the cup as you do the movements.

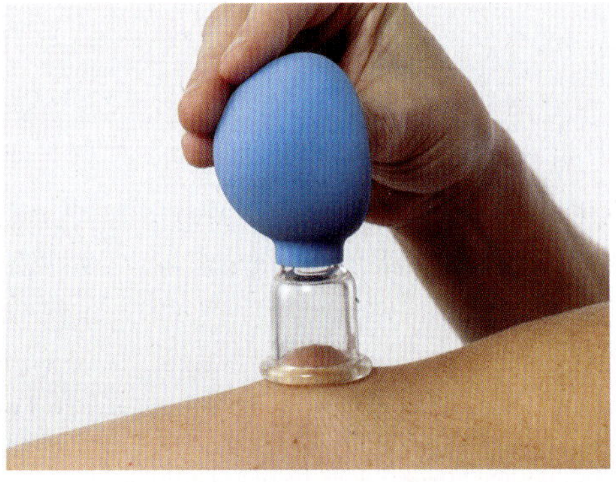

And while pushing the cup across the body offers similar effects, the greatest benefit comes with the enhanced lift and stretch of a comfortably applied cup as you move it along.

You do not want the skin in front of the cup to get backed up in front of the moving cup; ideally, the lifted moving cup is the highest point as you move it. (See images on previous page and above.) Do not lift so much that it detaches from the body; simply attach the cup, then lightly pull it upward from the skin as you begin to move it. Both you and the recipient should be able to feel this when you are doing it correctly.

CUPPING 101

A moving cup should slide with ease and be comfortable for the recipient. If this is not possible, consider using the lift-and-release technique to facilitate moving a cup. Also consider using the lift-and-release technique over any "speed bumps" while trying to move the cup smoothly along any line of movement. Never force a moving cup; rather, address any restricted tissue obstacle as needed with lift-and-release until it softens with cumulative treatments.

SUCTION PRESSURES WITH MOVING CUPS

Apply only light to medium suction pressure when moving the cup; otherwise, you can damage the soft tissues. Moving cups are more about the lift and manipulation of the cup in your hand and less about the strength of suction. There is no need to use stronger suction when doing these cupping treatments.

Using lighter suction pressure and lifting the cup as you work will allow for safe, effective applications without harm.

You should never feel any "ripping" or "tearing" as you move the cup. If you or the recipient feel anything like this, stop using the movement. Consider using lighter suction to move the cup, or the lift-and-release technique.

We discuss optimal suction pressure on page 57. For now, know that each person is different, but keep the pressure light to start.

The Morse Code of Cups

Moving cups are the most popular and easy-to-use technique, but many people make one common mistake: If the cup pops off at any point, they go back to the starting point and restart that line of movement. That is not correct!

That "pop off" could be a restriction (such as a tight muscle) or an anatomical "speed bump" (such as a bony ridge) that needs to be addressed where it lies. Therefore, for optimal results, each line of movement needs to be finished once you have started it. Don't overthink it; simply continue the line of movement to the end point, using whatever technique works best. This is where what I call the Morse Code of Cups comes into play.

Line of Movement

Line of movement refers to where you move the cups during the cupping treatment process. Each step addresses a certain part of the body. For example, for *Step 3: The Jawline* in the face-cupping treatment, you will move the cup from the center of the chin (the starting point), following along the entire jawbone progressing toward the ear (the line of movement), ending in front of the earlobe (the end point). To address the entire face, you will use a cup across every inch of the face, one line of movement at a time.

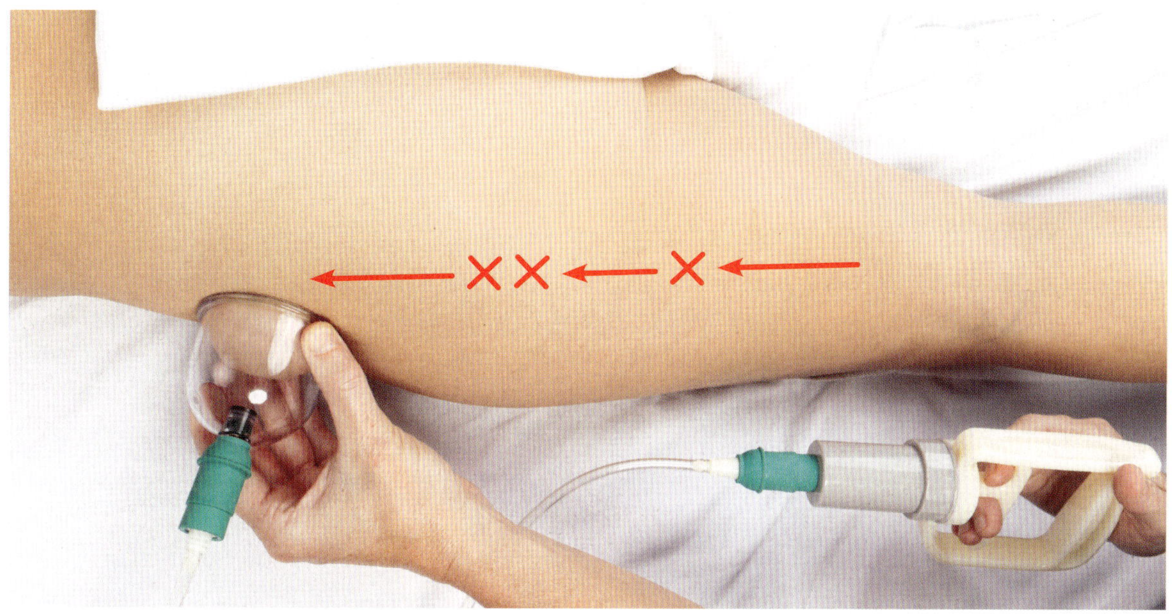

THE MORSE CODE OF CUPS
Demonstrated along the back of the thigh.
Arrows for moving cups, X for lift-and-release as needed.

DID YOU KNOW?

Morse Code is a method of communication that uses a series of dots and dashes. The Morse Code of Cups technique uses both the lift-and-release (dots) and moving cups (dashes).

The Morse Code of Cups is a combination technique of lift-and-release and moving cups. Once you get comfortable with the techniques and the concept of this treatment, it will become a very natural way of using the cups. It can be used along any line of movement, anywhere moving cups are not easy or not comfortable for the recipient. For example, the first few passes along a leg can be sensitive. Using the Morse Code of Cups will soften the line of movement, potentially allowing for easy moving cups within that same treatment or, as the results accumulate, at the next treatment. Alternatively, use this technique if you encounter a bony ridge "speed bump" that lies within the line of movement, as when moving a cup across the forehead or over the shoulder blade.

OTHER TECHNIQUES TO CONSIDER

There are so many techniques available for doing cupping bodywork. The few mentioned here are best for both cupping treatments mentioned in this book. For the Wrinkle-Reduction and Cellulite Focus options, there are a few additional techniques available.

- **Twisting** is just as it sounds: as you move the cup, twist it either back and forth or side to side. This technique is great for breaking up adhesions and adding a nice, stimulating sensation.
- **A two-cup tension hold** works to stretch muscles and fascia in opposite directions. This technique will work best for wrinkles, especially between the eyebrows in *Step 6* when focusing on glabellar lines in the forehead.
- **Stationary cups** are the most typical method of application when it comes to cups and the ones most responsible for creating cupping marks. In this book, stationary cups are used only as an additional option for stubborn cellulite dimples if more focused treatment is desired after using the other techniques. If choosing to apply a stationary cup, be sure to limit the length of time to less than a few minutes and monitor for any client feedback of discomfort.

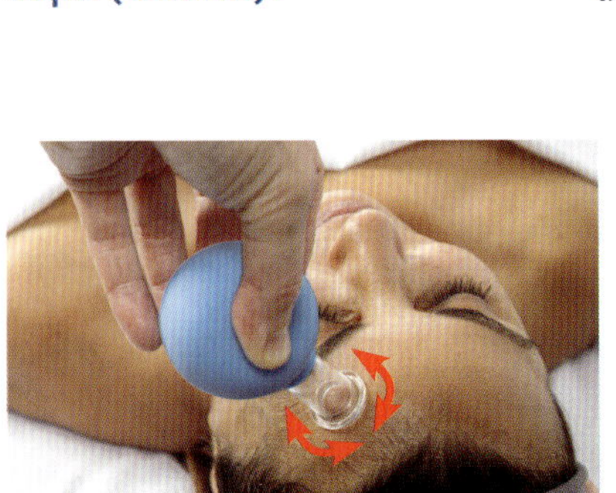

Twisting

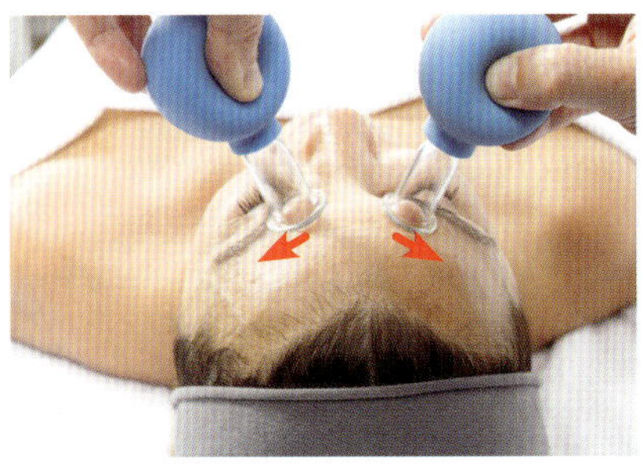

Two-cup tension hold

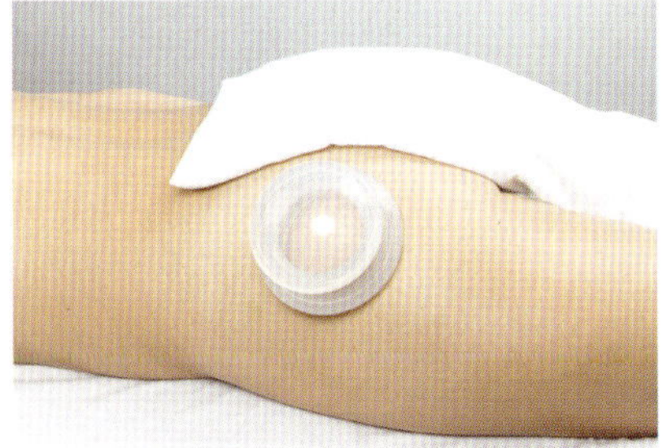

Stationary cup

Keys to Ensuring the Best Cupping Treatment

A few key elements contribute to optimal cupping treatments; the most important are sufficient lubricant, techniques used and suction pressure. Other elements that ensure efficacy include proper cup size choice, the pace of application, following the correct direction of lymph flow and using repetitive movements (without overdoing it).

SUCTION PRESSURE

While every person has a different sense of what light pressure means, remember that these cupping treatments are meant to address the most superficial layers of soft tissue. There is no need to use strong suction pressure! Do your best to use lighter pressure for these treatments—especially for the face cupping. The lighter pressure works every time and yields all the amazing results.

For face cupping, the good news is that most face cups have a maximum suction when you squeeze them, and that maximum is typically safe for face cupping.

I recommend testing the suction pressure on the upper chest or arm before you approach the face. First, try squeezing the cup just a little and attaching it to the skin to see how it feels. Then squeeze it as much as possible so you feel the difference.

Even though most face cups can provide lighter suction, it could still be too much for some people (if they are dehydrated or have thinner skin composition). Be sure to use whatever lighter pressure moves easily and feels the best for the recipient's skin.

For body cupping, however, there are no cupping sets that restrict the suction pressure to only the lighter pressure used in the body treatments in this book (unless you invest in a cupping machine with maximum pressure regulation).

Be sure to establish for each individual a light suction pressure that will ensure their comfort and ease of movement without pain or discomfort. Remember that lighter suction pressure is most effective in treating the superficial anatomy involved in cosmetic applications.

PRESSURE CHECK: CELLULITE REDUCTION

While lighter suction pressure is recommended for the body cupping treatment, using slighter stronger—medium, at most—pressure may be helpful over stubborn cellulite regions (see page 108).

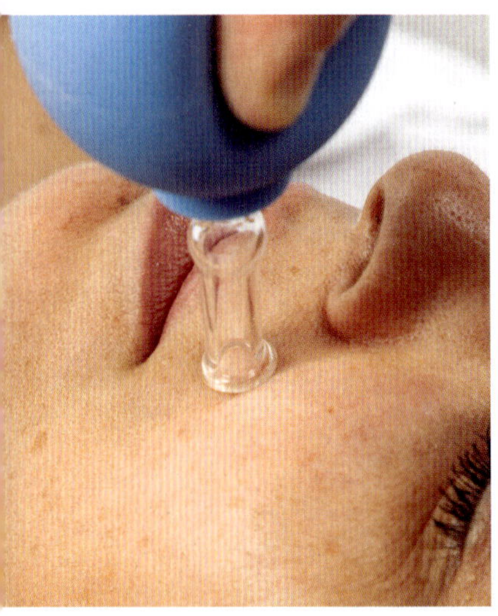

PROPER CUP SIZE

The intention with these cupping treatments is to affect as much of the general area being treated as possible, and not to focus on any one spot.

On the face, the small cups should be used in regions such as the upper lip and around the eyes, ensuring control of suction in smaller and more delicate spaces. The larger face cups will disperse suction over the skin and therefore are less likely to produce cupping marks.

For the body, be sure to work over any treated area with a larger cup relative to the body part. For example, the upper arm will require a smaller cup than the back, where a larger cup is better.

PACE OF APPLICATION

The speed and pace with which you move the cups can cause different reactions, too.

Moving cups at a slower pace is better for following lymph drainage pathways. Using cups slowly is best for longer, draining movements to efficiently encourage circulation. However, do not take too much time to do this treatment, as it will then not be as effective at influencing circulation of the entire body. While focus areas may take time, adjust your pace and repetition of passes as needed to ensure the timing is within reasonable parameters (see below).

Moving cups at a faster pace is better for stimulating focus areas. Faster moving cups can be used to energize tissues or break up areas of congestion, especially when focusing on cellulite. See page 182, where Cellulite Focus Options are detailed.

- For the face-cupping treatment, any technique used should be applied slowly across the face—nothing too fast or vigorous. Even for the wrinkle-reducing options, the pace will be relatively slower, so the delicate tissue integrity remains intact. While a relaxed pace is ideal, the movements should not be too slow, either. *The entire face treatment should take approximately 20 minutes.*
- For the body-cupping treatment, the pace will be slower along the drainage pathways and faster when choosing to focus on areas of cellulite. Again, don't be too slow, either. *The entire body treatment should take approximately one hour.*

PRESSURE CHECK: FAST-MOVING CUPS

Working at a fast pace is more likely to cause a sensitive reaction and can easily border on painful, so be sure to use lighter suction pressure the faster you go.

Make it a rhythmic application. Once you get the hang of it, maintaining an even, rhythmic pace creates a uniform method of application over every section and the entire part of the body being treated. Especially when working down the front of the neck, a slower, rhythmic pace ensures all the nerves and circulatory vessels remain undisturbed. And overall, an evenly paced, rhythmic application will feel good.

FOLLOWING THE DIRECTION OF LYMPH FLOW

Both cupping applications detailed in this book follow the movement of lymph along its pathways and within the watersheds of lymph drainage. For that reason, you must follow the step-by-step directions as they are shown and in the order in which they are written. The lymphatic system works as a closed circuit, one-way drainage system that has a very specific, sequential order of draining the body.

Additionally, most of the lines of movement described in this book follow the shapes and contours of muscles for lengthening and softening of wrinkles, or across common areas of tension to offer cosmetic benefits. While some advanced applications may differ from what is described here, this book is written for the general population. Following the instructions for application will offer the best, universal benefits for all.

REPETITIVE MOVEMENTS

As with most types of bodywork, repetition is necessary for both efficacy and general feel-good benefit. One pass over the area is an introduction, two passes get things moving, three to five passes complete the process! However, beware of overdoing it.

The total number of passes calculated for the face-cupping treatment in this book, including the additions of any wrinkle-reducing options, will ensure optimal results.

Since the skin over the rest of the body is not as sensitive as the face, it is possible to increase the duration of application to other body parts. We can add more passes with Cellulite Focus Options. Still, do not overdo it.

Regardless of what is suggested, always monitor for overworking the area. Indications of overworking include redness (more than pinkness), palpable heat (more than a subtle warming), and especially if the recipient reports pain or discomfort as the cupping continues. All are signs that no more cupping should be done for that person, in that session.

FAQ

WHEN ARE YOU "DONE" CUPPING AN AREA?

I always encourage cupping bodyworkers to *feel the tissue with their hands* and assess the area—first before using cups, then again after. They'll be able to feel a difference in temperature, texture and pliability indicating that the area is "done" being cupped.

However, I also caution them *not* to overwork any area. Ambition can sometimes override logic when you see how quickly change can occur. Remember that most compromised tissue didn't just happen overnight, so respect the cumulative process in all bodywork.

TECHNIQUES TO AVOID

What About Cupping Marks?
(What Not to Do)

Oh, the million-dollar question of cupping marks. One of the most common questions I hear is about those eye-catching, bruise-resembling cupping marks potentially appearing.

While cupping marks are common responses to stronger, more clinical applications on other parts of the body, there are many therapeutic benefits available from cups that do not mark the skin at all, especially in these two cupping treatments.

Obviously, when you are doing face cupping for cosmetic purposes, cupping marks are to be avoided. For this reason, the face-cupping techniques recommended here are the only methods of application that you should use.

Additionally, watching the skin as you do this treatment will allow you to see how the skin is responding. You can then adjust as needed. For example, one of the primary indications to stop cupping an area is if the skin starts to get red. While some pinkness to the skin is welcome—it indicates stimulated blood flow—redness can indicate overstimulation of the capillaries in the dermis, resulting in vascular microtraumas, which can produce those cupping marks.

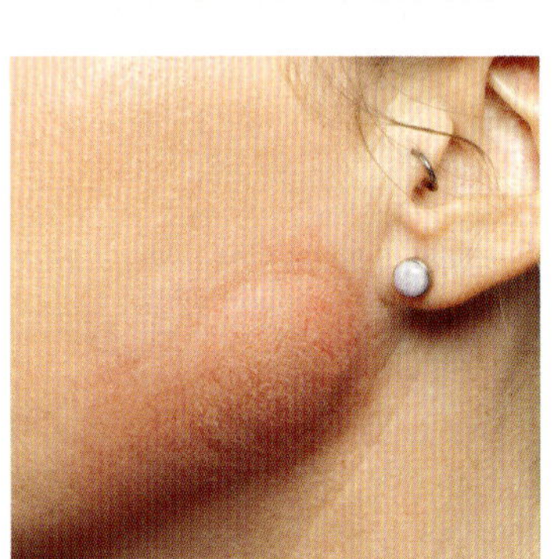

**CUPPING MARKS
ON FACE**

WHAT NOT TO DO

- **Do not use insufficient lubrication.** This is the first thing to check before you begin cupping, because it is that important for ensuring optimal treatment. Using a cup on drier skin will likely result in cupping marks.
- **Do not use strong suction pressure.** Lighter pressure is all you need for the face- and body-cupping treatments described in this book. Use comfortable, easy-to-move suction pressure to avoid cupping marks. Strong pressure not only makes it hard to move the cup, but it can be painful and cause cupping marks.
- **Do not use an inappropriate cup size.** Size matters for these cupping treatments. Using the largest cup available for any location will safely address more surface tissue for greatest efficacy, evenly dispersing suction pressure across the area. For example, you have to use your smallest cup in the upper lip region but using your smallest cup across

the cheek may result in cupping marks, so be sure to switch to a larger cup for the cheek. Likewise, using the largest cup possible when cupping the gluteal region will lessen the likelihood of cupping marks while also covering more surface area than a smaller cup.

- **Do not force a moving cup.** At any location where your moving cup meets resistance, there is a reason to stop. It could be not enough lubrication, or a tight muscle or a bony ridge. Check lubrication, or simply revert to lift-and-release over these areas to avoid cupping marks.

- **Do not use stationary cups.** For these treatments, there is no reason to park a cup anywhere. Stationary cups are known for leaving cupping marks. For the face cupping, even when we discuss suggested applications for TMJD (see page 81) or working into wrinkles, any of these more focused options do not use stationary cups. And with the exception of one Cellulite Focus Option, stationary cups are not recommended for the body treatment either.

- **Do not overwork an area.** If you do too much cupping across the same line of movement, chances are high that the skin will begin to show cupping marks. For this reason, always follow the recommended number of passes for each line of movement. Also, don't overwork wrinkled areas or cellulite dimples. Cupping is known to release tension in muscles, which can also result in cupping marks. If you travel across wrinkled or tight areas (such as the forehead or jaw), anything more than the recommended three to five passes could result in cupping marks.

Understanding Cupping Marks

For better or for worse, the possibility of cupping marks exists with any cupping treatment.

As soon as cups are attached to the skin, they take effect with negative pressure. And with this applied negative pressure comes both a pulling of the skin and tissues, which could cause tissue damage (the microtraumas discussed in *Chapter 1: The Science of How Cupping Affects the Body*), as well as the potential of "vacuuming out" any interstitial debris lodged within the many layers of soft tissue, both of which can result in those familiar cupping marks.

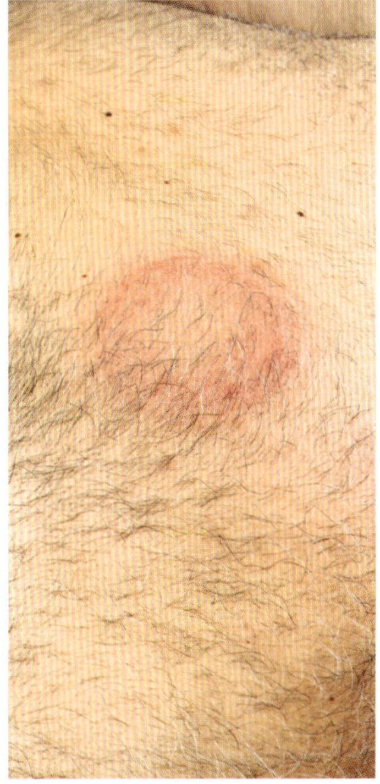

**CUPPING MARKS
ON BODY**

FAQ

CAN ALL SKIN COLORS GET MARKED BY CUPS?

While some skin tones may show marks more than others, the answer is yes, every color of skin can get marked.

Remember that a little goes a long way!

The subject of cupping marks has been widely studied, and there are many opinions on why they occur and what they are composed of. In some instances, alternative research has shown that cupping marks consist of interstitial debris, metabolic waste and "toxins" that lie stagnant within the layers of tightly woven, densely compressed connective tissues, that have been been "vacuumed" out from wherever they were embedded. Once released, this debris becomes visible in the more superficial layers of anatomy where lymph drainage occurs.

Additionally, cupping has been used to extract foreign materials from the body. These could be sutures from old surgeries, glass from motor vehicle accidents and even medications not fully metabolized. All sorts of materials can be vacuumed out by the application of cups.

Additional research has shown that cupping marks are responses to microtraumas and low-grade tissue damage, and different levels of blood disbursement result in the marks we see.

The necessary microtraumas discussed are, in fact, therapeutically beneficial, with the emphasis being on the micro-, not the macro-. The beneficial microtraumas are responsible for collagen and elastin production, the neovascularization to produce more capillaries and, on a larger scale, they help break up the adhesions involved with soft tissue dysfunction, including cellulite.

However, if cupping is done too strongly or aggressively, it can cause macrotraumas in the body. These can be painful and damaging, in the same way as a punch from a fist is a quick application of strong, aggressive, positive pressure to the body, resulting in a bruise.

Knowing this, you can understand why the potential for cupping marks depends on the intention and method of application.

POSSIBLE CAUSES OF CUPPING MARKS

Bodyworkers should be especially aware of the following possible causes of cupping marks.

- Overworking the tissue, which can result in excessive microtraumas and potentially more harmful capillary damage. This can occur anywhere you work more deeply into muscles to alleviate tension patterns.

ON THE FACE

- If the guidelines are not followed as suggested (ample lubricant, light suction pressure, no forced moving cups or stationary cups, etc.)
- Any focused cupping, whether on wrinkles or tension areas such as the jaw. These have the potential to create cupping marks, since the underlying muscle tension contributes to such areas of concern.

ON THE BODY

- If the general cupping recommendations are not followed
- If a location is overworked. For example, if a cellulite focus area is overworked in any one session, cupping marks will likely occur. These will likely look less like a circle and more like red speckling or light bruising over the area that was cupped.

Remember that all cupping bodywork is cumulative, and one session will not eradicate all wrinkles or cellulite.

What If You Do Get Cupping Marks?

One of the reasons this book came to be is because so many people were doing face and body cupping for cosmetic purposes incorrectly. If all suggestions are followed, cupping marks are unlikely to occur.

However, if any cupping marks do appear, they should not cause too much alarm. While they may be unsightly, cupping marks fade within a few days at the most, and the skin will look as it did before without any adverse changes.

The face is highly vascularized (meaning it has a high concentration of blood and lymph vessels), so the process of dissolving a cupping mark will happen quickly. And if any cupping marks appear over cellulite focus areas on the body, you can reassure your client that they are the results of necessary microtraumas that help break down those "dimples," and they will disappear in a few days.

Remember, true cupping marks should not be painful, but they are always a possibility when working with cups.

ANATOMY FYI

Most bruises take approximately ten to fourteen days to heal. If cupping marks do occur from excessive usage, they may similarly take several days to be fully resolved.

If bruising occurs during treatment, do your best to learn from it and trust that the skin will recover without issue.

SAFE CUPPING PRACTICES

CONTRAINDICATIONS

FAQ

CAN WE DO THESE CUPPING TREATMENTS IF SOMEONE IS PREGNANT?

While the face cupping is perfectly safe to do, this style of body cupping is contraindicated during pregnancy. While there are some wonderful cupping applications to enjoy during pregnancy, such applications are more advanced with and emphasis on safety during such vulnerable times as pregnancy.

SAFETY POINT

Use caution when working in and around endangerment sites (see following pages).

When using cups for bodywork, it is important to acknowledge some key safety points before you get started. In this chapter, we consider some contraindications to cupping, including endangerment sites as well as cosmetic injections and recent surgical procedures.

Specific Contraindications

- Never use cups over open wounds.
- Avoid using cups over any contagious skin conditions (such as chicken pox, herpes blisters) or topical irritants (for example, poison ivy, unknown rash).
- Never apply cups directly over bulging or herniated discs, or any severely compromised joints (for example, a sprained or dislocated knee).
- Avoid using cups directly over the belly button, as this is an open orifice into the body.
- Avoid using cups directly over any site of acute inflammation or recent injuries (sprains, strains, fractures).

SAFETY PRECAUTIONS

- Use lighter suction over any superficial vascular areas (such as the pectoral region, front of neck).
- Use caution when working in the abdomen.
- Avoid scraping the cup over any bones, as this can be painful.
- Use caution with anyone taking medications. Consider the contraindications noted for each medication and adapt the cupping treatment accordingly. For example, blood thinners compromise the circulatory system, so you should avoid strong or prolonged cupping, as bruising and/or tissue damage can occur more easily.

DERMAL CONSIDERATIONS

- Avoid sliding the cup over any raised moles or skin tags; cups could hurt or potentially tear the skin.
- When working with eczema, psoriasis, atrophic dermatitis or other skin conditions, exercise caution when using cups over any areas that appear inflamed, red, peeling or cracked.
- Avoid working on new tattoos; wait at least one month to consider working over the area.

ENDANGERMENT SITES

There are specific locations on the body, appropriately called endangerment sites, that require a cautious approach when it comes to cupping. These locations contain nerves, blood and lymph vessels that are closer to the surface, making them more vulnerable to damage with any bodywork or cupping.

- For the face and head: the *anterior triangle* and the *temporal region*
- For the rest of the body: the *axillary space*, the *femoral triangle* and the *popliteal fossa*

Anterior Triangle

The front of the neck—from ear to ear, jawline to collarbones—contains one of the body's most vulnerable endangerment sites, generally referred to as the *anterior triangle*. This region contains many vital blood vessels, lymph nodes and nerves, including the common carotid arteries, jugular veins, many cranial nerves (including the hypersensitive vagus nerve) and several clusters of delicate lymph nodes. It should therefore be approached with a lot of caution when doing face cupping.

Note: *The only technique to use in this region is the lift-and-release and using light suction pressure only. Never using moving cups and never use strong suction pressure here.*

Research has shown that any strong suction or aggressive cupping techniques could harm the delicate anatomy located in the front of the neck. The wrong method of cupping could cause damage to nerves located here, or to vital blood vessels, which could potentially lead to a hemorrhagic stroke. I often refer to this region as a "no-slide zone."

Additionally, cups in this region should be worked only in a downward direction: down the neck, toward the trunk. Since the lymphatic system is easily influenced, working in the opposite direction could redirect lymph fluids, drawing them into the head, causing congestion or headache.

ANATOMY FYI

The front of the neck is commonly called the anterior triangle, but technically there are two triangulated sections of vulnerable anatomy here: the posterior triangle and the anterior triangle. Both endangerment "triangles" contain many nerves, arteries, veins, lymph nodes and glands. They are generally referred to as the anterior triangle due to their location at the front of the neck, as "anterior" means closer to the front.

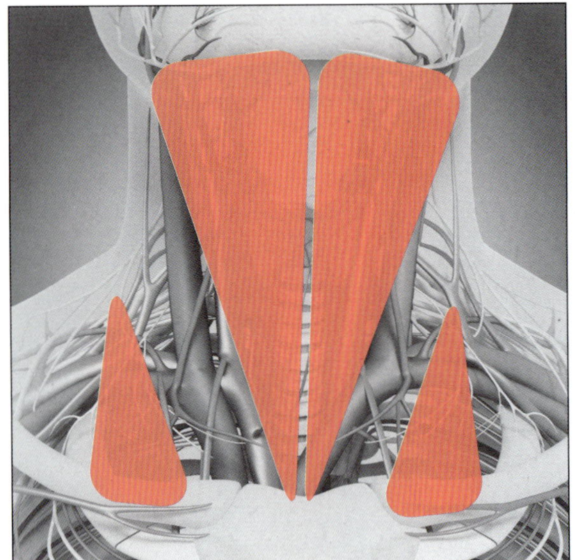 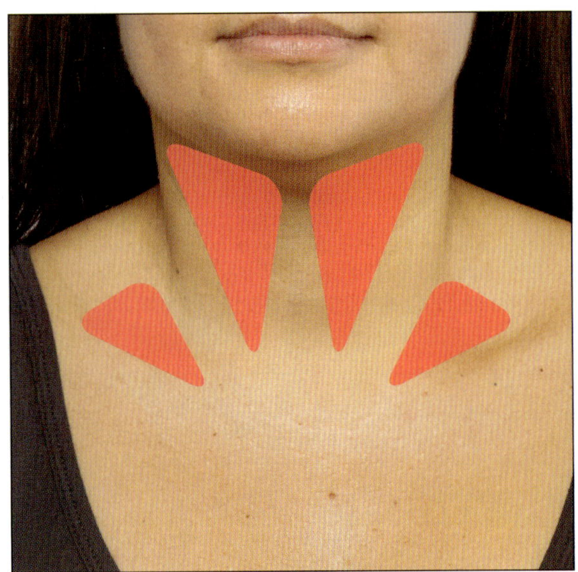

ENDANGERMENT SITES IN THE FRONT OF THE NECK (THE ANTERIOR TRIANGLE)

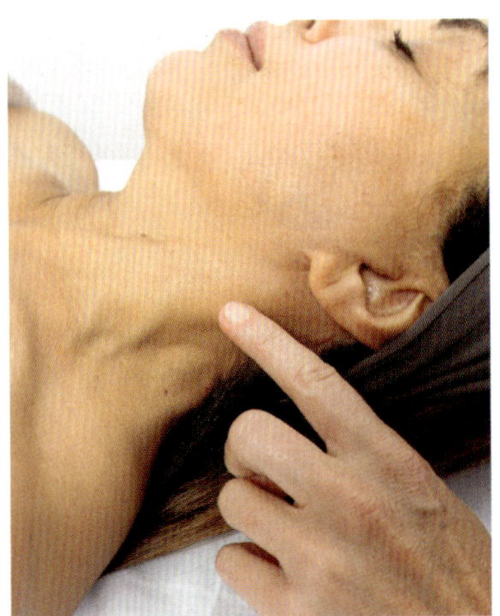

Visible blood vessels around the sternocleidomastoid (SCM) muscle

You will, however, travel down through the anterior triangle area many times during the treatment, since it is important to stimulate all the lymph nodes throughout this region. At the beginning of *Chapter 7: Face Cupping Step-by-Step Treatment*, you will learn how to safely work through this area. We will identify the exact line of movement down the neck, and the "jump-off" location from the face where you will always return to lift-and-release along the specified, exact lines of movement through this endangerment site.

While some may think cupping through here is unsafe, I assure you when you follow the guidelines outlined in *Chapter 7*— with or without a cup—everything will be perfectly safe and effective.

Temporal Region

Located between the hairline and the outside edges of the eyes is a small endangerment site known as the *temporal region,* commonly called the temple area or temples. There are important blood vessels and nerves located here, so caution should be used when working through this area. The temporal region includes the temporal arteries, temporal veins and the trigeminal ganglion, which divides into three nerve branches that innervate the face. The preauricular lymph nodes are located in front of the ear, just below the temporal endangerment site.

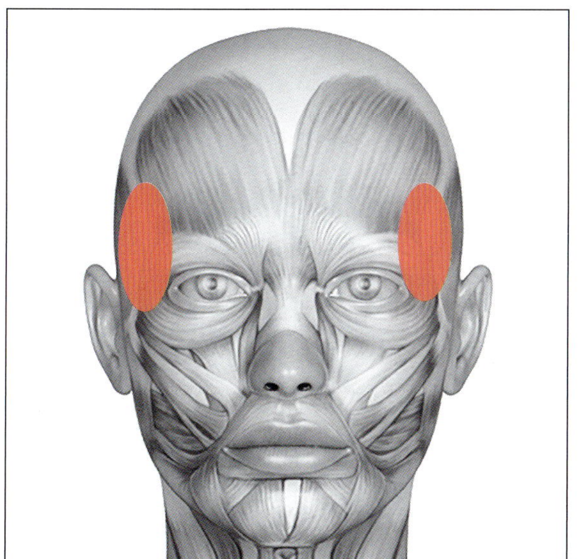
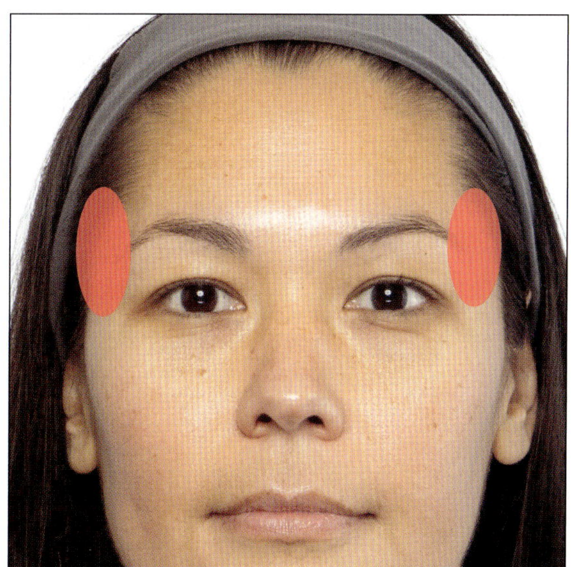

TEMPORAL REGION

Every person has different skin, some thinner or more fragile than others; in this region some blood vessels may protrude on some people while on others they are barely visible. If you encounter veins that bulge here, detach the cup as you approach the area—in *Step 6* for the forehead, *Step 7* for the eye and *Step 8* for the eyebrow—and skip over them, then reattach the cup and continue the line(s) of movement.

Again, to keep the treatment safe and comfortable, do not use strong suction or stationary cups in this common endangerment site.

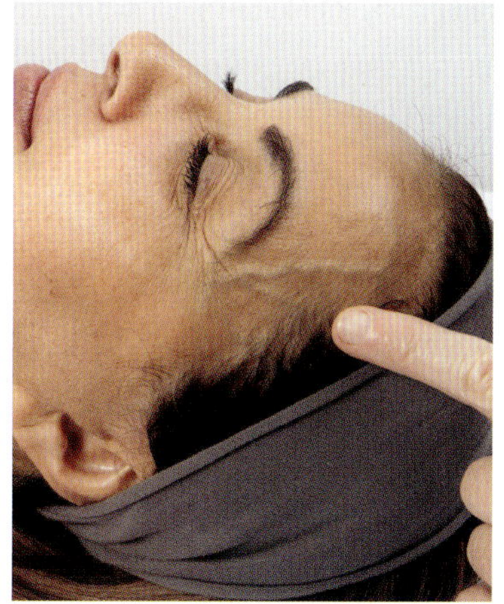

Visible blood vessels in
the temporal region

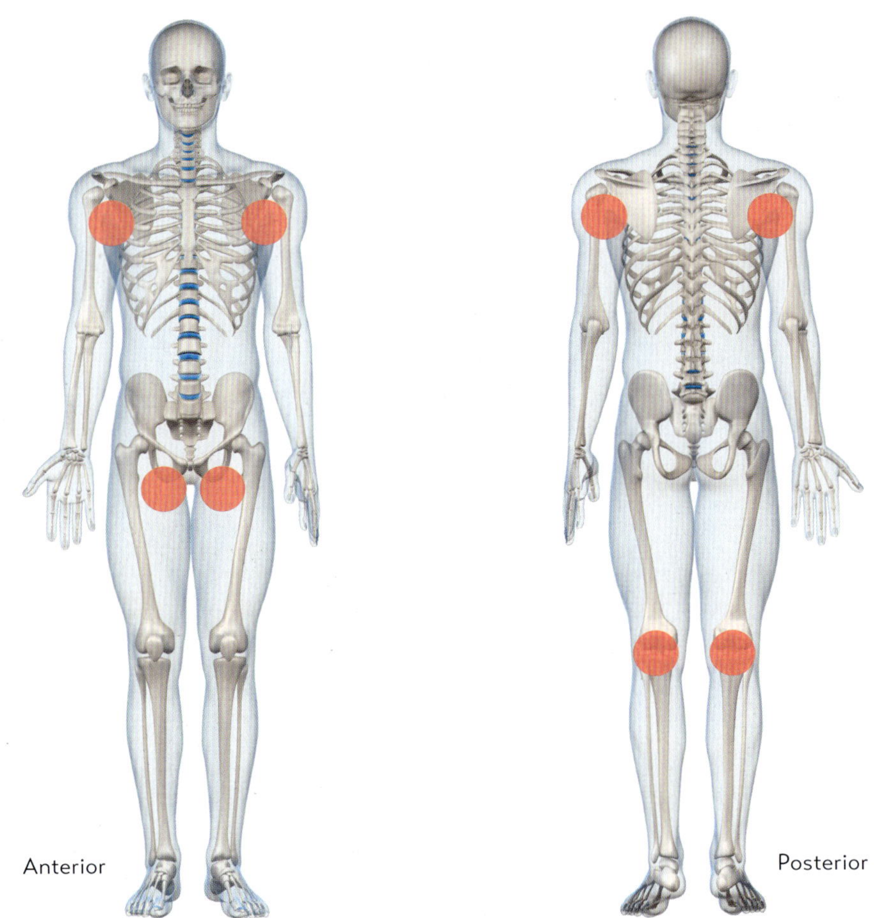

ENDANGERMENT SITES OF THE BODY
The axillary space, femoral triangle and popliteal fossa

Axillary Space

The *axillary space* is found where the arm meets the torso in the area commonly called the armpit. There are many lymph nodes, blood vessels and nerves located here. This area contains the brachial arteries, the basilic veins, segments of the brachial plexus (specifically the ulnar, median and musculocutaneous nerves) and several clusters of lymph nodes.

Femoral Triangle

The *femoral triangle* is located at the top inner thigh. Commonly known as the groin area, this location contains the femoral arteries and veins, the femoral nerves and three divisions of the inguinal lymph nodes. It is also a very personal area, since it is located directly next to the genital region.

Popliteal Fossa

The *popliteal fossa*, an area of the leg located in the soft tissue space behind the kneecap, is another vulnerable site. It contains the popliteal arteries and veins, the tibial nerve and a cluster of popliteal lymph nodes.

In *Chapter 10: Body Cupping Step-by-Step Treatment*, there are instructions on how to stimulate lymph nodes in each of these endangerment sites. Considering the sequential flow of lymph, gently addressing the lymphatic activity for this treatment is necessary—yet it must be done with great caution. Any strong suction pressure or vigorous movements of cups could harm the many nerves, blood and lymph vessels located within each of these regions.

In many hands-on methods of bodywork, these endangerment sites are avoided or barely manipulated to ensure their safe keeping. One of the few types of bodywork that works directly in each of these regions is manual lymph drainage, with its very light, positive pressure. For this reason, there is a Cup-Free Option for each site in case you choose to stimulate these lymph nodes with your hands only.

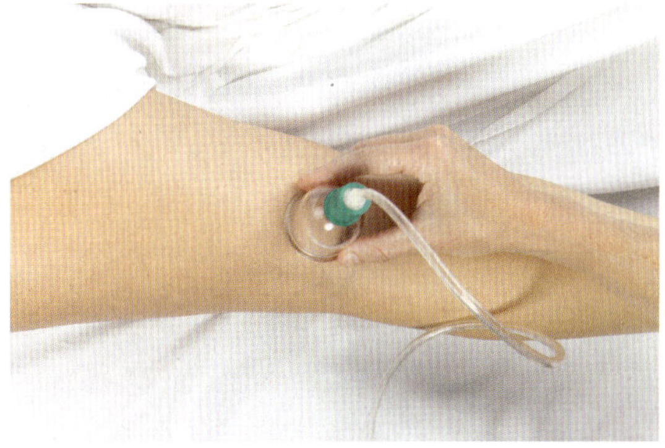

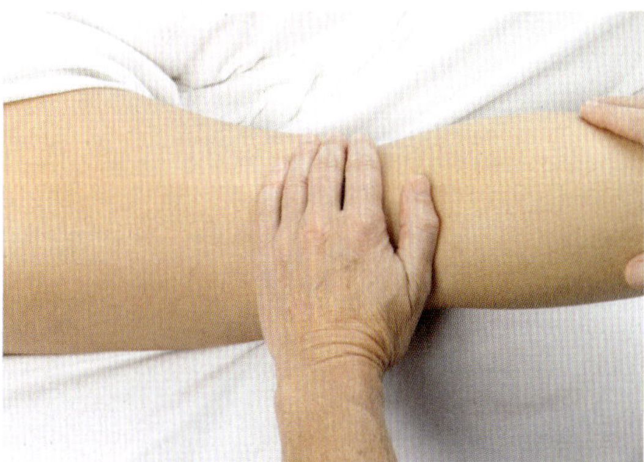

Stimulating sites of lymphatic activity with and without cups

WORKING WITH COSMETIC INJECTIONS

For more information about other injectable materials in the body, see page 85.

Cosmetic injections are widely available today for many different, cosmetically focused reasons. However, with cupping there are specific safety considerations to acknowledge. While there are all types of materials that can be injected into the body and the face—both cosmetically and medically—we focus here on cosmetic injections. The same rules and potential reactions apply to the body as they do for the face, since we are generally discussing the same injectable materials.

If any materials have been injected into the face area, you should avoid working over the entire face for approximately thirty days. This goes for any fillers or wrinkle-fighting materials.

Why? The material that has been injected is intended to stay exactly where it is. If you attempt to use cups over the area too soon, these materials will be dislodged from their intended locations and begin to travel along lymph drainage pathways to other locations. For example, some cosmetic injections contain a modified neurotoxic protein that is intended to stay where it has been applied in order to block nerve conduction to a muscle, thus inhibiting muscle contractions that cause wrinkles.

While a neurotoxin is generally safe wherever it is injected, if it enters the circulation too soon, it could cause muscle weakness, nausea, vision problems, trouble speaking or swallowing, breathing problems or loss of bladder control. Any other injected materials (collagen, fat transfers, etc.) that are meant for cosmetic enhancement are also injected with location-specific intentions, so if you use cups too soon, you could move those materials elsewhere in the body.

After thirty days, the injected materials have been metabolized and thoroughly settled into the site of application, so chances are less that cupping will affect their intended use.

Just to be sure, travel over the area in question (forehead, cheeks, etc.) with lift-and-release only for that first session after the thirty days. This allows you to test how the local tissues respond, to make sure the injected materials don't irritate the skin when cupped, and so on, and ensures that the tissue isn't too sensitive for this initial, post-injection treatment.

POST-SURGICAL CONSIDERATIONS

Whether the person receiving treatment has had a small eyelid lift, a full facelift, a tummy tuck or liposuction, any surgical interventions should be left to fully heal for six to eight weeks before you attempt any cupping over or around the area.

Furthermore, no cupping should ever be done if there remain any scabs, sutures, significant bruising or raw tissue, as these are clear indications that the area is still healing and is too fragile for cupping.

Often, I encourage people who are having such surgical procedures to receive medical release from their surgeon to receive cupping bodywork. If their surgeon is not familiar with this manner of cupping, asking for medical release to receive an "invigorating massage" will suffice.

If there is a question or concern of safe timing, please do not attempt any cupping just yet!

Scar Tissue

While the focus of this book is cosmetic rejuvenation, with surgical alterations there will always be scar tissue to consider. The age of scar tissue (new or old), the location of the scars (on the face or in the abdomen) and the type of scarring (atrophic or keloid) all need to be assessed before attempting to work in the area. Here are some guidelines:

- If there are any scabs or raw tissue, cupping is absolutely contraindicated.
- If the scar or surgical procedure occurred four weeks ago, do not attempt the cupping treatment yet; wait six to eight weeks unless you are professionally trained in post-surgical cupping bodywork.
- If it has been more than eight weeks, you can most likely proceed with treatment. However, work on or around the scar lines with caution. I recommend using the lift-and-release with light pressure over new scars.
- If the scar is more than one year old, cupping across the area should be fine. Again, always check with recipient for any sensitivities; even scars that are many years old can retain pain and discomfort.

BEFORE BEGINNING CUPPING

ASSESSING THE SKIN

SKIN RESTRICTIONS

What about raised moles or skin tags? Avoid moving cups across them, as it will hurt or possibly tear the skin; use lift-and-release instead as you move through the area.

What about tattoos? Any new tattoos should be avoided for approximately thirty days to ensure full healing has completed. If scabs or sensitive areas linger, avoid cupping the area until it has completely healed. If unsure, consider waiting a few weeks longer. Since they are permanent works of art, ensuring their preservation during the initial healing phase is crucial. After that, cupping can be done over tattoos without issue.

In preparation for cupping, we must take inventory of the skin, thoroughly examining it to create the best possible treatment plan. Here we address many common exceptions which, if they apply to the person being treated, require adjustments to personalize the standard treatment process.

For example, for a face-cupping treatment, the average skin type requires the application of approximately a coin-sized amount of oil. For the full-body treatment, a few ounces are more than enough. If the client's skin is naturally hydrated, the moving cups will slide easily with these suggested amounts of lubricant. But if the skin is dry and dehydrated, they will need more of any applied product to have a successful outcome.

For cupping the face, there are recommendations on how to deal with facial hair, acne, sinus congestion and jaw tension (TMJD). For body cupping, exceptions can similarly be made for body hair and vascular concerns. There are also suggestions for working with loose skin, injections and any recent surgical procedures as well as information about scar tissue.

Although these are among the most common exceptions to be made when doing cupping bodywork, there are countless other conditions or individual needs that mean cupping will have to be adjusted accordingly to accommodate that person. In fact, there are far too many conditions to discuss in one book. For bodyworkers, it is ultimately up to their professional methods of assessment to decide who can or cannot be cupped.

This book and the material discussed are intended for the generally well person who can receive bodywork without considerable restrictions. If your client has any conditions such as rosacea, psoriasis, facial paralysis, fibromyalgia, or a history of cancer treatment that affect the body with symptoms that go beyond the benefits of cupping discussed in this book, consider seeking professional cupping bodywork services or receiving advanced training before attempting either of these treatments. For more information, see *Know Your Limits* on page 87.

CUP-FREE OPTIONS

For every step of the face-cupping treatment, and some of the body cupping, there are also recommended Cup-Free Options.

When you use a Cup-Free Option for the face, it is important to address the entire face and neck every time, so be sure not to skip any section of the face if the skin does not respond easily to the general cupping instructions. The Cup-Free Options are the best way to address any exceptional region without excluding it from the treatment.

Looking for a Cup-Free Option for the body? Unlike face cupping, this full-body treatment does not have as many cup-free options. Why? For the greatest efficacy, as much of the body as can be cupped should be cupped. Also, when it comes to full-body treatments, many of the reasons why a person cannot be cupped are also reasons why this treatment is not recommended for them.

Cup-Free Treatment Tips

- When choosing these Cup-Free Options, be sure to follow them as instructed for each step.
- For most of the Cup-Free Options, your fingers will be flattened and closed, contacting as much surface area as possible.
- Use light pressure only. The emphasis is on gently addressing the skin's surface only and with very light pressure. Working with this light, skin-stretching pressure will stimulate the underlying lymph capillaries, and the direction in which you move will further influence the lymph movement along its drainage pathways.
- Where half-circles are mentioned, the intention is to gently stretch the skin's surface with flattened fingertips in specific directions. Your fingertips are not sliding across the skin's surface; rather than slide, simply create a gentle stretch of the skin with these half-circles in the correct direction. These half-circles stimulate the underlying lymph capillaries for lymph movement along the same lines of movement you would use with a cup if you could.
- Around the eyes, there are other cup-free instructions for "tapping" beneath the eye and light "pinching" of the eyebrow rather than half-circles. These different techniques are best for addressing the delicate tissue around the eyes.

EXCEPTIONS

As you work through the face- and body-cupping treatments, you may encounter exceptional situations that will require a change in the basic methods of application, such as facial hair, acne, jaw tension, very loose skin, varicose veins or recent cosmetic procedures. Each of these common exceptions and how to respond accordingly is described below. There are also reminders on what to do with every treatment step.

Facial Hair

Cups can be attached to almost every naturally skin-covered surface of the body, but they attach best to well-lubricated, relatively hairless skin. When facial hair is present, that can make it difficult to create the sealed connection between the cup and the skin's surface, especially if trying to use lighter suction pressure over the delicate soft tissues of the face.

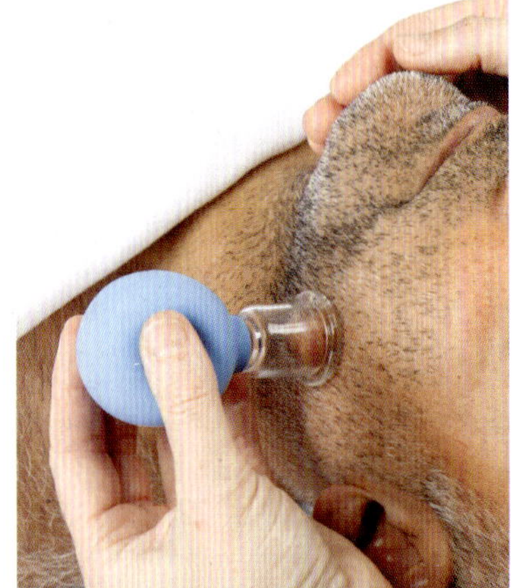

ADDRESSING FACIAL HAIR WITH A CUP AND SUFFICIENT LUBRICATION

While it is possible to cup over some body hair (see facing page for details), facial hair will usually not allow for cups to attach easily. Some facial hair can in fact be cupped, but you will have to judge according to the facial hair whether it will work or not. Has it been shaved recently? Is it a full beard or just a mustache? Is the hair thin and soft or thick and coarse? With an ample amount of applied oil, shorter, more recently shaved or sparser facial hair may allow for some lift-and-release applications or perhaps even some moving cups, but longer or thicker facial hair will not allow for a cup to attach at all.

The eyebrows should be addressed differently on an individual basis also, as the hair varies tremendously from person to person. A thinner eyebrow is easily cupped, while a thicker eyebrow cannot be cupped at all.

Do not skip over any hair-covered regions, especially the areas where facial hair tends to grow. There is a wealth of lymphatic activity over every section of the face, so it is best to address the entire face every time. Using the cup-free methods will ensure optimal results from the cupping treatment.

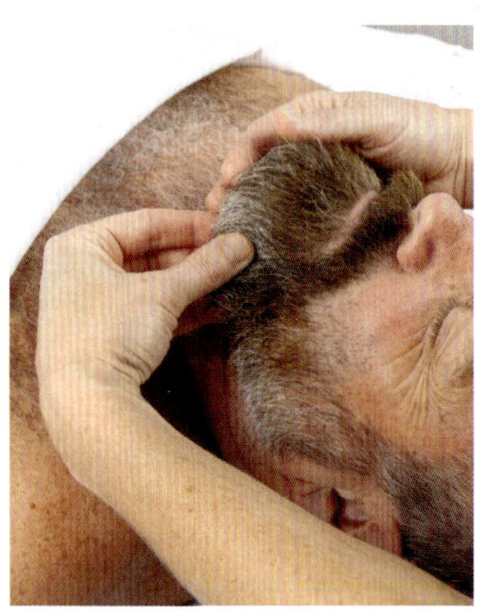

OPTIONAL PINCHING OF LONGER FACIAL HAIR

Recommendation: Follow the cup-free instructions recommended (*Option 1*), or use the alternative *Option 2* if applicable.

Option 1: Use your fingers to follow the cup-free instructions. These are described for every step of the treatment process.

Option 2: Gently pinch and lightly pull the facial hair as you progress along each hair-covered line of movement, following the same instructions as the other Cup-Free Options (starting points, lines of movement, end points and number of passes). This gentle lifting of the skin will mimic the lifting offered by the lift-and-release technique—and it feels great when done correctly! This option generally works best for thicker or longer facial hair (such as beards and mustaches).

Body Hair

There may be challenges when trying to apply cups over excessive body hair similar to those encountered when using cups over a face with facial hair. While an average person's body hair will not cause an issue, thicker or more coarse body hair that typically relates to male clients may require some adjustments, including additional lubrication and modified techniques.

Recommendation: Add more lubrication. You will most likely need more than the average recommended amount of oil applied over dense areas of body hair. Typical areas include the back, chest, legs and arms. Also, adding a lotion or cream to combine with the oil will provide a better medium to create the seal between the cup and the hair-covered area. While some people may have a better response to this combination of products than others, use your best judgment when deciding if this will work for your client or if you will not be able to use cups over their body hair.

Try modified techniques: If, even with the addition of more lubricant, body hair inhibits a cup from moving easily, use lift-and-release only over that area.

If these adjustments do not help, this cupping treatment will most likely not work for the individual.

Acne

Acne is a dermatological condition that affects a great number of people. It is characterized by inflamed or infected sebaceous glands in the skin, most identified by red pimples and blemishes on the face. Acne commonly affects hormonal teenagers, but it can also occur for many other reasons, such as poor diet, environmental exposure or inadequate skincare.

WHAT ABOUT BALD CLIENTS?

Bald clients have the added benefit of enjoying cups across the surface of the skull, too! In *Step 6: The Forehead*, there are options for treating the head of a bald client (see pages 144 and 149).

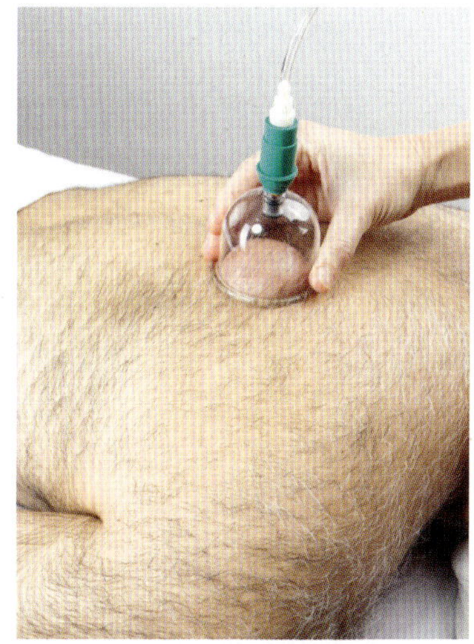

ADDRESSING BODY HAIR WITH A CUP AND USING SUFFICIENT LUBRICATION

FAQ

CAN I DO THIS FACE-CUPPING TREATMENT WHEN SOMEONE HAS A COLD OR FLU?

Do *not* do this treatment within the first 72 hours of onset of sickness. Why? In those first days, the lymphatic system works hard to produce immune-fighting cells to fight the infecting sickness. If these necessary excess fluids are cleared before ready, the body works even harder to replace what was prematurely cleared and could increase congestion or inhibit the body's infection-fighting ability.

After the first 72 hours, you should be able to proceed without issue—and help your client feel better fast!

Cupping may help to clear the congestion associated with nonhormonal acne, but you must work mindfully around pimples and acne spots. Try avoiding them and do your best not to "pop" them while you work, since that would create an open wound, which could allow blood to escape and/or bacteria to enter the skin.

If by chance you pop a pimple, clean the skin's surface immediately and thoroughly clean the cup, too. Never continue the treatment over the popped pimple, as that is now an open wound.

Recommendation: If you approach a pimple as you work, use the lift-and-release technique to skip over that spot. If an area has many acne spots, consider using the Cup-Free Options until the breakout has cleared.

Sinus Congestion

Relieving the congestion associated with sinus issues is one of the most popular benefits of face cupping.

Several locations in the face and head are more affected when sinus congestion is an issue, specifically around the nose, eyes, cheeks and forehead. These locations are collectively known as the paranasal sinuses.

As you work through each affected area, you may encounter some sensitivity if sinus congestion is an issue. If yes, be sure to work with comfort in mind and follow the recommendations accordingly. However, if no sensitivity occurs and congestion is a factor, the suggested therapeutic options can be added in as you work across the sinus areas in the cheeks, forehead and eyebrows.

Recommendation: Use the lift-and-release technique over any hypersensitive or congested areas.

Therapeutic Option 1: Add in a few more passes of lift-and-release to stimulate the area, enabling internal flushing mechanisms to clear congestion. The most common sites for this option are next to the nose in *Step 5* when treating the cheek, and in *Step 6* when treating the forehead near the eyebrow.

Therapeutic Option 2: After adding *Option 1*, applying a few more passes of a slowly moving cup across the affected areas in the cheeks and forehead will add some tension relief, and the sensation is easily experienced and appreciated.

Jaw Tension

The cheeks cover most of the jaw area, a large area that contains many muscles. Throughout the region are muscles involved with the temporomandibular joint (TMJ) and the muscles of the jaw, including the temporalis (above the ear), the masseter and pterygoids (both in the cheek) and digastric muscles (below the jawline).

Considering how much we use the jaw for eating and talking, this area can hold a lot of muscle tension. Accumulated tension here can contribute to muscle pain, headaches and dysfunction of the joint, commonly referred to as TMJD.

Often, there will be some resistance as a cup moves across the cheek and jawbone areas. If someone suffers from TMJD, this resistance will be even more obvious and palpable. Cupping works well to help alleviate this tension, so if this is an issue for your client, add in the suggested therapeutic options as you work across the cheeks.

CLINICAL SUGGESTION

If you work specifically with people who have TMJD issues, consider offering the entire face-cupping treatment *after* the more focused jaw therapy is completed. This will support lymph movement from the area and relax the client who may have experienced discomforts often associated with more therapeutic manipulations of the jaw.

Cupping Marks Possibility

As you work to address tense muscles, the possibility of cupping marks exists. The more you work into jaw tension, the greater the possibility that cupping marks may occur, because the cups are breaking up muscle tension patterns, which can lead to the speckled cupping marks on the surface skin. Also, considering the tissues of the face are among the most sensitive of the entire body, they are also the first to show cupping marks if any focused cupping is applied.

While this is an unsightly result for many, cupping marks will disappear within a few days, leaving some much-needed TMJ muscle relief. Keep this in mind and monitor the skin for any redness while you work. If redness becomes obvious, that is a good indication to finish addressing the TMJD issues for that session. A little goes a long way here, so don't overdo it!

Recommendation: If you encounter any "speed bumps" along the way, do not force the cup to move across it. Instead, simply revert to the lift-and-release technique to get across that section. Thereafter, you can finish that line of movement with another moving cup, employing the Morse Code of Cups combination technique (see page 55) or simply finish that line of movement with lift-and-release.

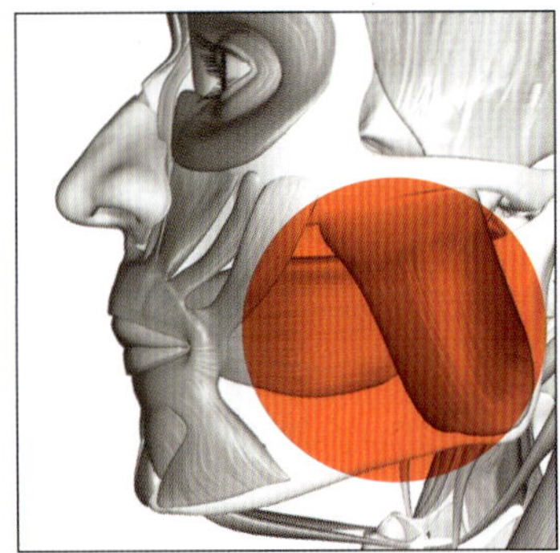

TMJ region

FAQ

WHAT IF VERY LOOSE, THIN SENIOR FACE SKIN?

As we age, the supply of collagen and elastin diminishes, and the older we get, the thinner the skin in the face becomes. While you can offer this treatment to seniors—I have clients in their 80s who enjoy this treatment—working with more caution is imperative. Lift-and-release is generally the only technique used with seniors, as moving cups can be difficult on extremely loose and brittle skin.

Or simply follow the Cup-Free Options so your older clients can still receive the benefits of this face treatment.

To address TMJD issues, consider the following options:

Therapeutic Option 1: As you work across the cheeks, any "speed bumps" can be treated with a few extra lift-and-release placements in each location before continuing along the designated line of movement.

Therapeutic Option 2: Twisting and rolling the cup here are great options. As you encounter speed bumps in the jaw area, slow down and gently address the tight muscles.

- Slowly twist the cup back and forth over the tight muscles.
- Gently roll the (attached) cup around over the surface of the cheek to stretch and manipulate these muscles. If you find this hard to picture, think of how a tossed coin rolls on its edges before it settles.
- You may consider adding a little more suction—medium suction is plenty—and make the twisting or rolling techniques slower, penetrating deeper into the jaw muscles instead of just addressing the skin's surface. (You wouldn't do this where the goal is wrinkle reduction.)
- With either therapeutic option, consider also lifting the cup away from the face as you work for an even deeper therapeutic effect. The lift stretches the muscles here with negative pressure—and it feels great!

Caution: You should not see the delicate eye tissue move while you apply any of these therapeutic options, nor should you pull the lips outward toward the ears. If either of these occurs, use less suction pressure and make sure you are not straying from the TMJ cheek and jawline areas.

Loose Skin

Loose skin can occur for many reasons and can affect any region of the face, most commonly along the jawline. It can also affect the body, especially the upper arms, midsection and thighs. If loose skin does not allow for an easy-to-slide moving cup, follow the recommendations here so you can treat the entire face and body without skipping any areas.

Recommendation: Use the lift-and-release technique to address the lines of movement across areas of very loose skin. With time and subsequent treatments, the skin will tighten up, indicating improvement, which will progressively allow for smooth moving cups and safe tissue-toning.

If the skin is extremely loose, consider using one hand to treat the area with the cup, and the other hand to hold skin taut as you slide the cup along. This two-handed method of application anchors the loose skin as you move the cup along the designated line of movement; it is meant to be gentle and supportive. Be sure the skin is not pulled too tightly if you choose this option. With time, the skin should tone up and the assistance of the second hand will not be needed, but it is useful to help create a more accessible, flat surface for the cup to attach to easily when needed.

Vascular Concerns

One of the most common concerns with cupping involves vascular health. While it is important to clinically evaluate each client before cupping and to use your professional expertise accordingly, any vascular issues require specific attention when cups are involved. Of the many possible considerations, the two most common are varicose veins and spider veins, which generally affect the legs.

Varicose veins are large, raised, swollen blood vessels that can be seen through the skin or palpated as vascular abnormalities. Caused by a weakening in the blood vessel wall or from faulty valves, its symptoms may include pain, cramping, circulatory congestion, lethargy, restlessness, burning, tingling and heaviness.

Since cups take effect with negative pressure, any added lift of the tissue over a varicose vein will only cause more damage to the affected blood vessels. *If varicose veins are present, cupping is absolutely contraindicated for that area.*

Recommendation: If varicose veins are present, there are two primary options: working around the area with cups or following cup-free recommendations.

Option 1: Work around the area with cups. If there are only a few varicose veins present, using the cups on other parts of the leg should be safe. It is best to work above and around the site of varicosity; this will be beneficial to supporting the regional circulation. Be sure to have sufficient lighting in the treatment room to see the area and use your hands to feel for any raised or deficient vascular pathways.

SAFETY FIRST

Deep vein thrombosis (DVT) is a potentially life-threatening condition involving blood clots that, if manipulated, could dislodge a clot and send it into circulation, possibly making it to the heart or brain and causing fatal results. DVT is an absolute contraindication for body cupping as well as general bodywork.

If someone has a history of DVT many years ago, chances of such potentially dangerous results are less likely. Yet no matter the history, be sure to get medical approval before considering any body cupping treatments. With DVT, this is a universally understood precaution for bodyworking professionals.

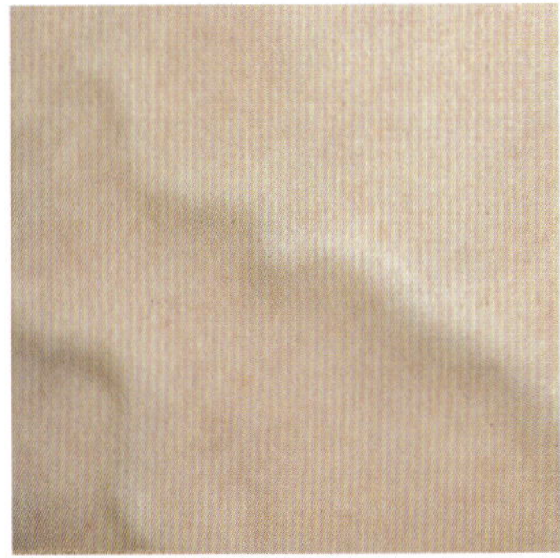

VARICOSE VEINS

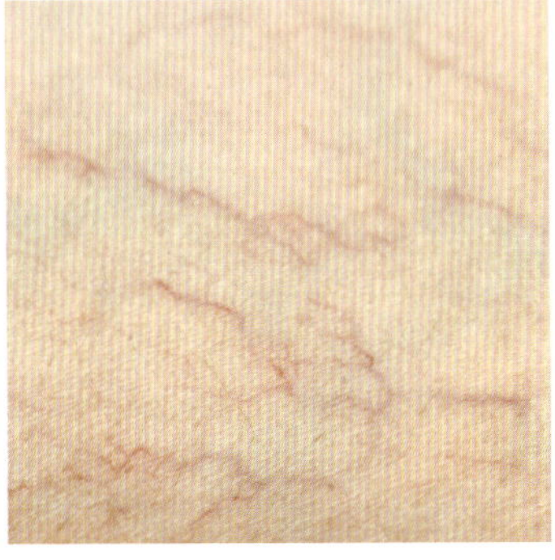

SPIDER VEINS

Note: If varicose veins are involved or in the same area as spider veins, do not use cups over the spider veins.

Option 2: If there are many varicose veins present in any area, use your hands only to follow the lines of movement lightly. While there may be a wish for body cupping to reduce unsightly cellulite dimples or poor circulation, varicose veins always override the decision to use cups.

If there are too many veins to use your hands over the site without discomfort, this treatment is probably not suitable for the person.

Telangiectasia, or spider veins, are a mild version or early onset of varicose veins. They are caused by unhealthy valves inside feeder veins, resulting in blood pooling and nonfunctional, "dead end" veins that are visible under the surface of the skin. In addition to concerns about appearance, some discomfort may be experienced. Since these microtraumas in the smallest segments of the veins are not as compromised as varicose veins, gentle and light-pressured cupping may be applied. Be sure to use very light suction pressure over any spider veins, and always travel in a centripetal direction—toward the torso—to support optimal venous return for these challenged vascular segments.

Recent Cosmetic Procedures

There are many options for people seeking the assistance of professional cosmetic enhancements for the face and different parts of the body. No matter what procedure has been done, cupping is still beneficial, yet for the best outcome we must proceed with timing and caution in mind. Since there are major differences between injections and surgical procedures, they are addressed independently here.

INJECTIONS
For the face

Regardless of the material injected, wait approximately thirty days before attempting this face-cupping treatment. After thirty days, the injected materials have been metabolized and settled into the site of application, so chances are less that cupping will affect their intended use.

Recommendation: During that first treatment—after thirty days—use lift-and-release only across the sites of injections. If the skin is sensitive to that technique, switch to Cup-Free Options for these areas. At the next treatment (a few days later or thereafter), try lift-and-release again and, if not sensitive, proceed with whichever technique you prefer.

For the body

Cosmetic injections: Injections into the body vary from what is typically done for the face. Still, there are procedures to enhance parts of the body (such as the gluteal region) via injection rather than implants. If the injection is related to cosmetic procedures (as with neurotoxins, collagen fillers), the same rule of waiting approximately thirty days before cupping applies.

Non-cosmetic injections: Other injected materials should be considered at the time of treatment, too. For example, insulin injections should remain undisturbed for several hours after being administered. Also, hormone injections or other materials injected for systemic circulation (such as vaccinations) may be sensitive to cupping for a few days after injection. If you are unsure how to proceed with injected material, follow the thirty-day rule, consult with a professional trained in this area or seek advanced training in cupping bodywork.

Recommendation: After thirty days, use lift-and-release only across the sites of injections during that first treatment. If the skin is sensitive to that technique, switch to Cup-Free Options. If the injection site is not sensitive to lift-and-release, proceed with whichever technique you prefer, keeping in mind the client's comfort.

COSMETIC SURGERY

No matter what the surgical procedure, the skin, circulatory system and muscles have all been affected and need time to heal. Some of the most common cosmetic enhancement procedures include implants (such as breast or gluteal implants), reductions (such as breast, loose skin or tummy tucks), alterations (such as facelifts) and liposuction. The average waiting time after any surgical procedure before you can consider cupping bodywork is approximately six to eight weeks. Recent cosmetic procedures are discussed in *Chapter 4: Safe Cupping Practices*; please review that information if needed.

For more details about injections and surgical procedures, please revisit *Chapter 4: Safe Cupping Practices.*

SAFETY POINT

Still have questions? Please check with your client's cosmetic surgeon for when they can receive body cupping or an "invigorating massage." While most hands-on manual lymph drainage therapies can begin shortly after surgical procedures, cupping affects the body in a totally different manner. Alternatively, consider working with a trained professional for that first body-cupping treatment to get started in the right direction. Or perhaps invest in advanced training for post-surgical cupping applications.

FAQ

CAN CUPPING HELP WITH STRETCH MARKS?

Striae, otherwise known as stretch marks, are a form of scar tissue formed by rapid stretching or distortion of the dermis. This damage to the skin directly affects the collagen, elastin and general cellular formation in the affected area. Stretch marks come in many sizes, colors and consistencies, can occur over most surfaces of the body (the abdomen, hips, legs and chest) and, while commonly caused by pregnancy, they can occur for many other reasons, including rapid weight loss or gain, medications or genetic or pathological conditions.

We have seen many positive and lasting results with reducing the appearance, texture and tone of stretch marks, yet, just like any other line of scar tissue, they never totally disappear. Considering the positive effects cupping has on every element of the skin, it can't hurt to try and see!

The concern regarding surgical procedures is more about recent procedures, rather than those done years before. For example, if someone had a facelift, breast or gluteal implants several years ago, you should be able to follow a general treatment plan without issue. However, be mindful not to work too aggressively over the implant—for example, in the case of a gluteal implant, when a foreign object is permanently attached—if trying to break down any cellulite. Similarly, if someone had a tummy tuck done years before, this treatment should be perfectly safe to receive without exceptions being made. Since cupping through the abdomen is universally done without strong pressure or vigorous movements, the older scar tissue and underlying visceral organs in abdomen will remain undisturbed.

SCAR TISSUE

With every surgical procedure comes scar tissue. Cupping for scar tissue is very beneficial, but at the same time requires a higher level of training than this book can address. Be sure to avoid using cups on any newly forming scar tissue until the site is completely healed; anything within approximately one year from the procedure is considered a new scar. Never use cups if there are any scabs, sutures or raw tissue at the site. While it is generally safe to follow the basic recommendations made here when the time is right, each individual person must be clinically assessed. Every person's recovery is different, and there are many different types of scar tissue to consider. Cupping over newly formed scar tissue before it has properly healed could not only hinder the healing process, but it could also create worse, more complicated scar tissue. If unsure, do not use cups; consider seeking assistance from a professionally trained, post-surgical cupping practitioner.

Recommendation: When the time comes (approximately six to eight weeks post-op), for the first treatment post-surgery, use lift-and-release only to test how their skin will respond, especially close to any site of incision. If there are any areas that are sensitive, uncomfortable or visibly irritated by the cup (for example, if the scar line looks vulnerable), switch to the cup-free recommendations until things feel better. It takes time to heal and, while it may be frustrating, it is in your client's best interests to wait until the skin is ready.

KNOW YOUR LIMITS

With any bodywork, there is only so much that can be addressed in one book, and the same goes for cupping and its benefits. For the face, we discuss the use of cupping for cosmetic benefits as well as benefits for TMJD muscle relief, sinus congestion and post-surgical considerations. And for the body, we explore cupping for cellulite reduction and contouring, and its benefits for muscle relief, circulation challenges and additional post-surgical considerations. Since both treatments follow general lymph drainage pathways, they can offer much benefit to the generally well person being treated. And while the directions may look simple, there are many instances that may cause you to pause and ask questions.

There are so many other, more complicated pathological conditions that affect the face and body for which cupping could offer great benefits; however, more advanced training is required to do so safely. For example, dermatological conditions such as rosacea, cystic acne and psoriasis can receive benefit, as well as more pathological conditions such as headaches, Bell's Palsy and even head traumas (including concussions and cranial surgery).

For the body, there are countless instances where the basic cupping described in this book should not be applied. For example, special consideration is required for clients who have history of cancer treatments, especially if they have received radiation, had lymph nodes removed or are experiencing lymphedema. The same goes for treating an individual with more pathological conditions such as fibromyalgia, lupus or scleroderma. And, as with any bodywork, restrictions associated with medications need to be acknowledged; for example, people taking blood thinners will most likely bruise and sustain soft tissue damage if cupping is applied in some of the invigorating manners described in this book.

The techniques described in this book are intended for people who are generally in good health and recommended for use by professional bodyworkers. It is up to the trained bodyworker to know more about any pathological condition, to understand exactly what cupping offers and to know how to adjust accordingly for the best outcome of the client. Moreover, when a client has exceptional needs beyond your experience, you must be aware of your limits.

Those of you who use cups for self-care should also follow these guidelines when assessing how to treat yourselves.

SAFETY FIRST

In bodywork, two common sayings are "do no harm" and "when in doubt, refer out." There is no shame in referring to a specialist in such cases. Again, this book focuses on many of the wonderful benefits cupping offers, but advanced applications deserve advanced training.

OTHER TREATMENTS AND CUPPING

WHAT ABOUT EXFOLIATION TREATMENTS?

Exfoliating is very beneficial to overall skin health. There are many different products and tools that can be used to exfoliate the skin (from sugar scrubs to microdermabrasion); some can be gentle while others, however, are quite invasive.

If choosing to combine exfoliation with cupping at the same treatment time, any of the gentler exfoliation treatments should be fine. While it is generally recommended to do cupping *after* the gentle exfoliation has been completed, some may choose to do cupping *before* gentle exfoliation for greater product absorption; practitioners are encouraged to experiment accordingly.

However, I recommend you avoid combination, same-day cupping treatments with any of the stronger, more aggressive methods of exfoliation.

If you are a practitioner who combines hydrotherapies or uses other tools in treatments, such as guasha scrapers, kneading devices or needling, there are a few additional considerations to acknowledge.

Hydrotherapies

If choosing to combine hydrotherapies that use hot or cold temperatures (such as saunas, steams, hot tub soaks, ice therapies) the same day as either face- or body-cupping, I recommend you use warming treatments before cupping, and perhaps consider cooling treatments after cupping. Why?

Anything warming will improve circulation and soften the skin, offering a more pliable area to be treated. A steam towel to the face is a nice pre-treatment, as is a sauna or a soak for the body.

Anything cooling, however, will constrict and restrict, which is the opposite of what cupping will do to the soft tissues. This can be both counterproductive and uncomfortable. There are some extreme cold applications that rapidly boost circulation (for example, cryotherapy plunge pools), but in my experience, even that rush of blood does not result in the ideal soft tissue environment before any cupping.

See *After-Care Recommendations* on pages 162 and 240 for more about using any of these temperature-sensitive add-ons following the cupping treatments.

Cupping and Other Tools

For the face, I highly recommend that you do face cupping independently from other scraping or pressure-sensitive modalities, as it can simply be too much for the delicate face tissues. There are many great tools other than cups used to stimulate circulation, break down wrinkles and revitalize the face. However, if too much is done to this delicate skin at one time—no matter what the tool—the risk of overworking the skin exists, which could result in swelling, bruising or cupping marks.

For the body, it is equally important to do the body cupping as a stand-alone treatment. While the skin on the body may not be as sensitive as on the face, it can similarly be overworked with too many treatments done at once, resulting in bruising, cupping marks or pain.

Some professionally trained bodyworkers and skincare specialists may choose to proceed with combination treatments, using multiple tools during one session. If opting to use other modalities in conjunction with cupping, I highly recommend you experiment with the order of application to see what works best for the desired outcome. When doing so, consider the effects of boosted circulation, lymph drainage and negative pressure occurring at the same time. In my opinion, experience and the consensus of many cupping practitioners, offering these cupping treatments at the end of any combination program is the best way to leave the client's body in a revitalized and relaxed state of being.

If using needles or other treatments that break the skin is part of the intended treatment plan (as in microneedling, acupuncture, blading), do the cupping first, because the punctured skin is considered an open wound. Traveling over the area with cups will not only draw blood but could also introduce bacteria to the skin's surface.

Note: *Remember to allow 48 hours between cupping treatments so you do not overwork the body. For more information on treatment plans and frequency of applications, see pages 163 and 242.*

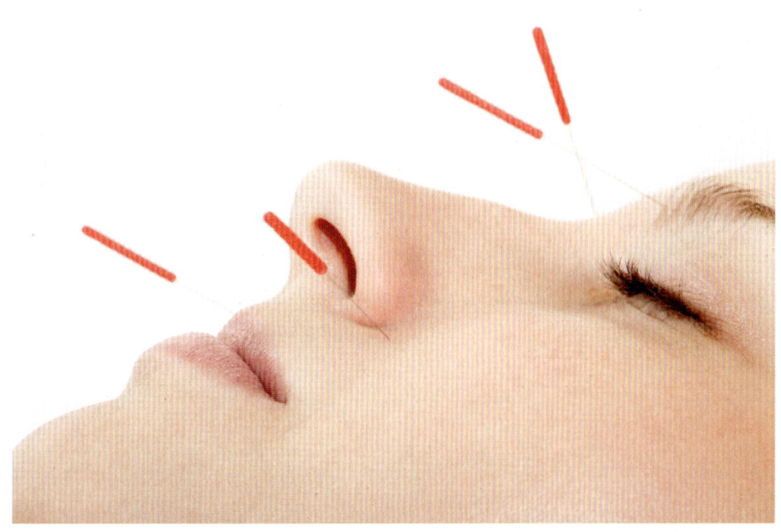

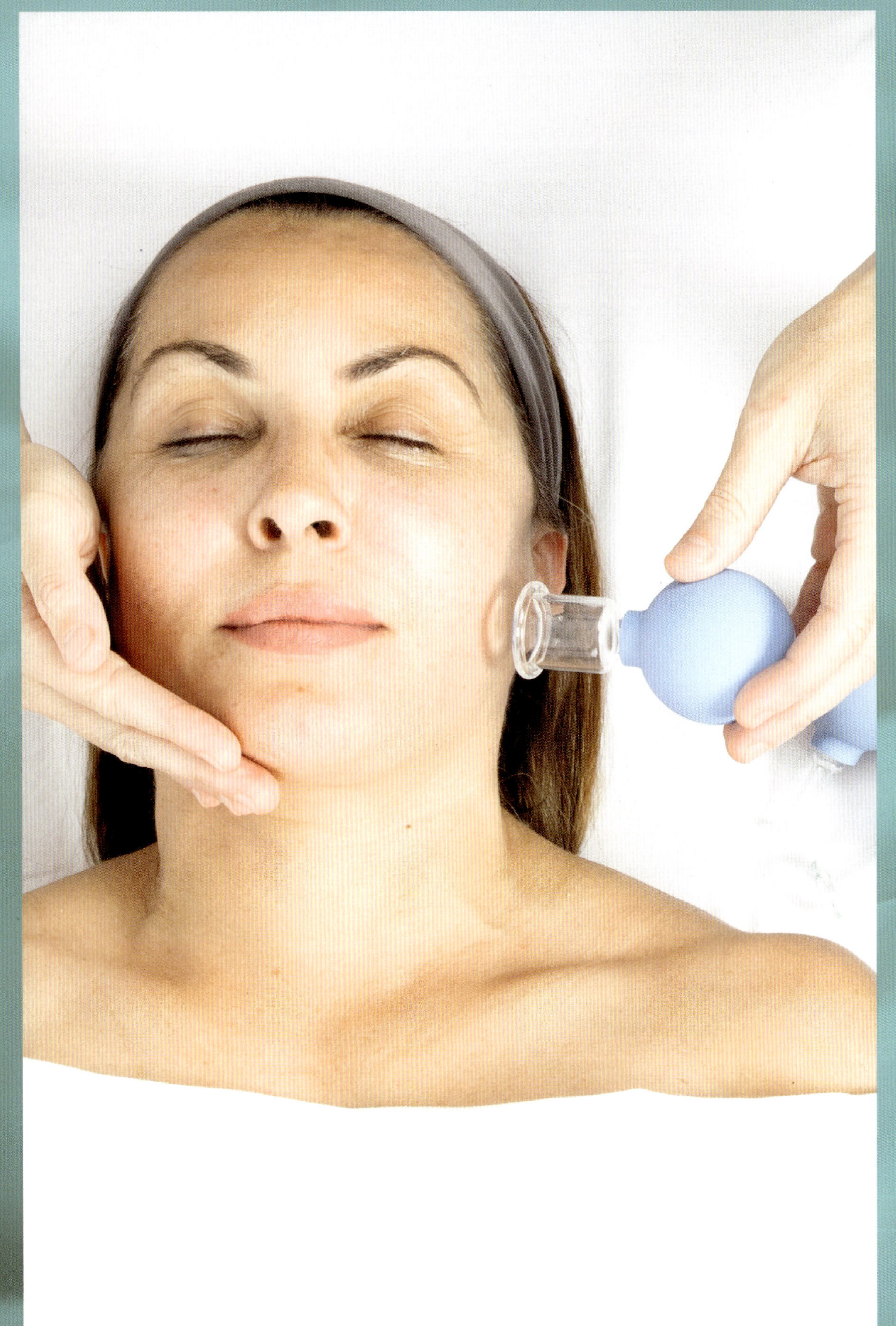

PART II

FACE CUPPING

CHAPTER 6

FACE CUPPING FOR COSMETIC REJUVENATION

ANATOMY OF THE FACE

The anatomy of the face involves many body systems, with the integumentary, circulatory and muscular systems being most notable for this discussion. (For more about these systems, see *Know Your Anatomy* on page 16 in *Chapter 1: The Science of How Cupping Affects the Body.*)

The face is generally the part of skin most noticed, and it contains some of the most sensitive surfaces of the body. While the outer layers of the skin are exposed and vulnerable to the elements, the inner layers are attached to the underlying muscles and fascia, with nerves, blood and lymph vessels woven throughout every layer.

The face is highly vascularized, which means there is a high concentration of blood and lymph vessels in the area. The face relies on optimal microcirculation and lymph drainage to maintain its health.

Even though it is small in size, the face and neck contain many muscles; of the more than 650 muscles in the body, the face and neck contain almost 50. Every facial expression requires several muscles and the nerves that activate them, making for a high amount of activity within a small region.

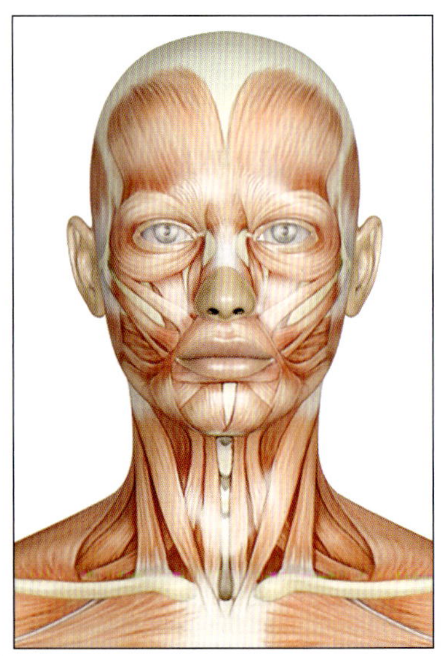

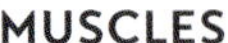

MUSCLES

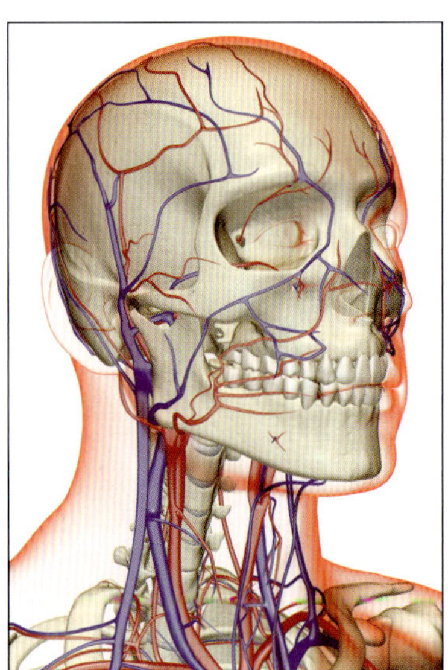

BLOOD VESSELS

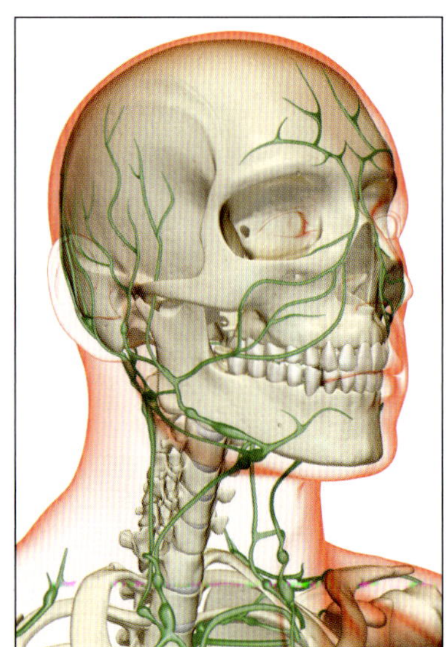

LYMPH VESSELS

WRINKLES AND WRINKLE REDUCTION

A wrinkle is a natural crease or line formed in healthy skin, resulting from the skin's loss of firmness and elasticity over time.

Some skincare specialists refer to wrinkles as *hyperfunctional facial lines*, due to the repetitive contraction of muscles during recurring facial expressions such as laughing, smiling, furrowed eyebrows or frowning.

Wrinkle formation has both intrinsic and extrinsic factors to consider.

Intrinsic factors are those we cannot control, such as aging. As we age, collagen production diminishes, fat cells start to shrink (causing skin to become thin and brittle), with eventual depletion of optimal circulation and skin integrity.

Extrinsic factors are those that we have influence over. These include smoking, exposure to free radicals and pollution, UV radiation exposure (from the sun) and repetitive muscle contractions associated with facial expressions.

These repetitive muscle contractions accumulate over time, forming adhesions that set into the skin, muscles and fascia. These internal adhesions attach and pull on the underside of the skin, thus creating the creases and indentions on the surface known as wrinkles.

As well as cosmetic concerns, muscular restrictions can also contribute to aches and discomfort anywhere in the body, even in the face. The most common sites of facial tension are in the jaw (temporomandibular dysfunction or TMJD), forehead and neck regions.

Healthy Skin Components

Beyond the physiological components of healthy skin, other contributing factors for total skin health include:

Optimal hydration. Every person should drink a good volume of water daily. While recommendations vary, some say drinking eight glasses of water daily is sufficient, while others suggest you divide your body weight in half and drink that amount of water in ounces. For example, if you weigh 140 pounds, 70 ounces of water daily is recommended.

Good nutrition. Countless resources including books and nutritional experts offer information on what a healthy diet is. While individual needs vary, a well-balanced, nutritious diet is important to maintain healthy skin.

Skincare regimens. A routine of washing, moisturizing and protecting the skin (using sunscreen) is equally important. Skincare professionals can provide personal suggestions.

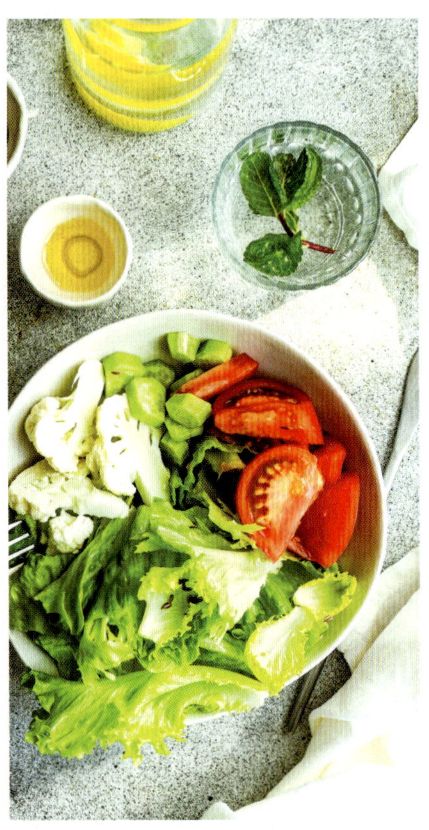

COMMON WRINKLES

With every facial expression, many muscles are involved. Some of the most common wrinkle-formations from facial expressions include:

- **Nasolabial lines.** Also known as smile lines, these form between the nose and mouth, usually tracing a diagonal line from the corner of mouth to the nostril. They are typically associated with smiling.

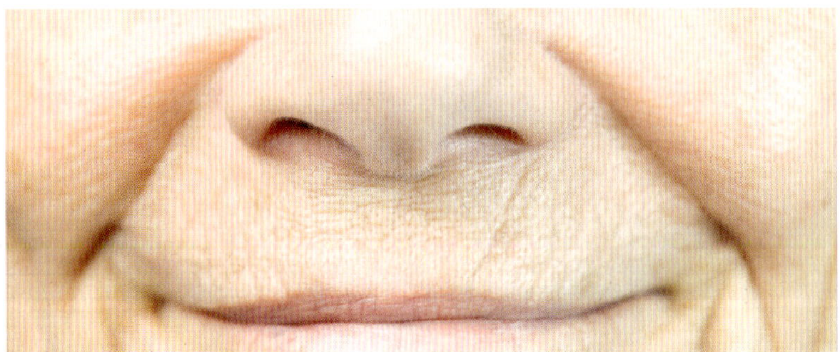

NASOLABIAL WRINKLES

- **Forehead wrinkles.** The creases that form across the forehead are typically caused from any facial expression involving raised eyebrows, including excitement, worry or joy.

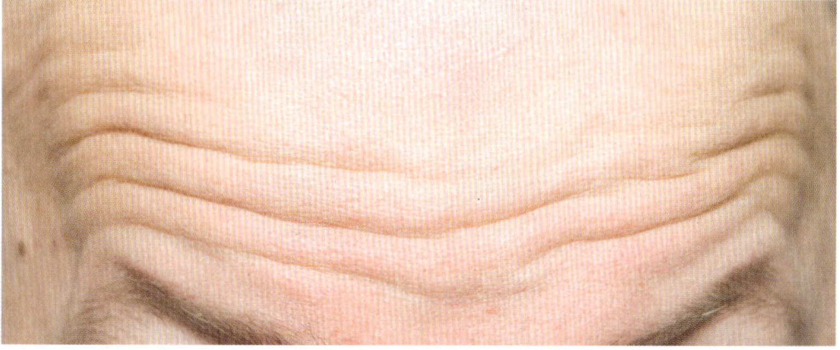

FOREHEAD WRINKLES

- **Glabellar lines.** Also known as the *11s,* these form between the eyebrows, at the top of the nose. They are typically associated with frowning, squinting or worried expressions.

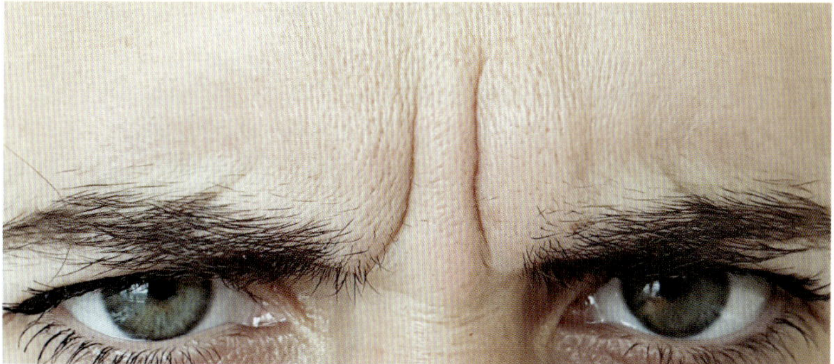

GLABELLAR LINES

- **Crow's Feet.** Also known as the other smile lines, these form at the corners of the eye, usually in a crescent-like pattern around the outer edges of the eye and top of cheek. They are also typically associated with smiling.

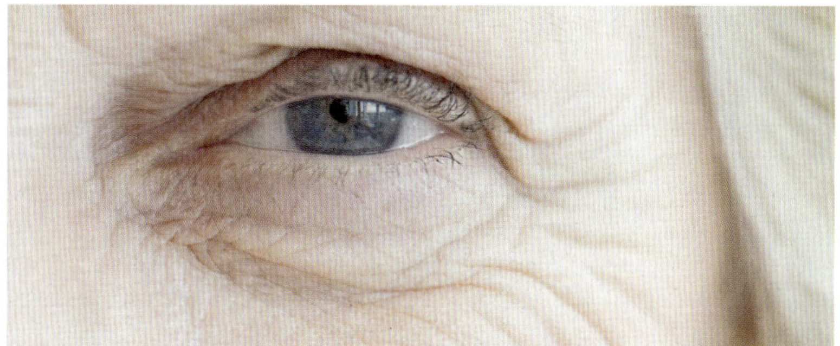

CROW'S FEET WRINKLES

WRINKLE-REDUCTION OPTIONS

In *Chapter 7: Face Cupping Step-by-Step Treatment*, there are Wrinkle-Reduction Options for these common wrinkles where they occur within the treatment process. If choosing to add these options, make sure to monitor for signs of overstimulation to avoid cupping marks during the treatment process.

POSSIBLE CUPPING MARKS WITH WRINKLE-REDUCTION APPLICATIONS

Cupping is one of the best noninvasive modalities for addressing wrinkles. Since cups lift the tissue with negative pressure, the outward stretch of the skin, fascia and muscle combined with the bodily fluids drawn into the area allows for some impressive reduction of wrinkles. Yet with this extraordinary benefit comes the potential for cupping marks.

As discussed in *Chapter 3: How to Use Cups*, cupping marks can occur anywhere on the body, especially in locations such as wrinkles. While the desire to immediately erase wrinkles is natural, face-cupping results are best when approached with realistic expectations. Yes, immediate benefits will be seen and felt, but remember that the wrinkles did not form overnight. The best results will come after several cumulative treatments. See *After-Care Recommendations* on page 162 and *Make a Treatment Plan* on page 163. Be sure to monitor for signs of overworking the area (such as redness, not just pinkness), and trust that the best results will take several treatments. If cupping marks do surface, they will disappear within a few days.

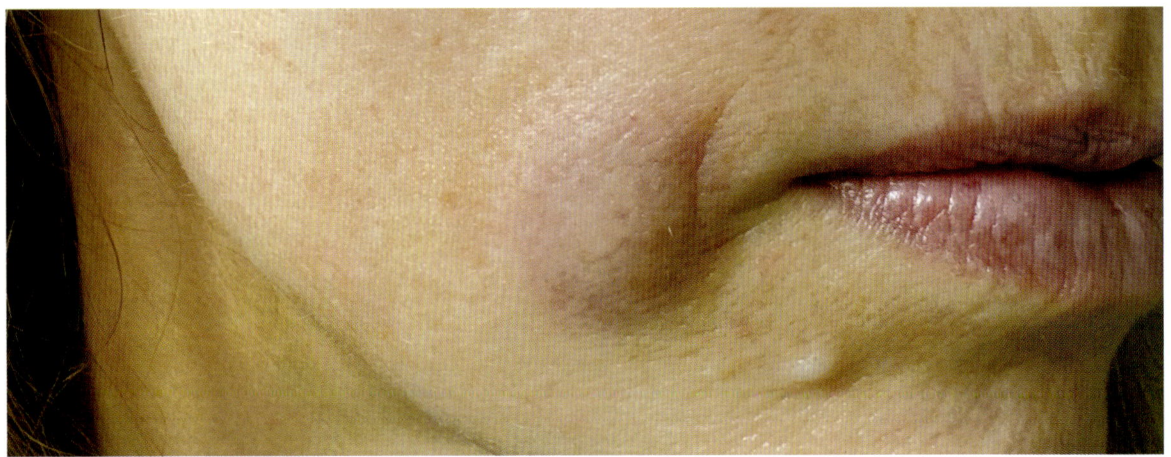

EXAMPLE OF CUPPING MARK RESULTING FROM FOCUSED
WRINKLE REDUCTION TO NASOLABIAL LINES

Aging Is Inevitable and Our Body Responds Accordingly

While each body system is affected with age, hormonal shifts also play a major role in how our body systems function.

Over time, the circulatory system slows down, which contributes to inadequate blood and lymph flow and decreases the production of cells that contribute to our skin's health, including collagen and elastin proteins.

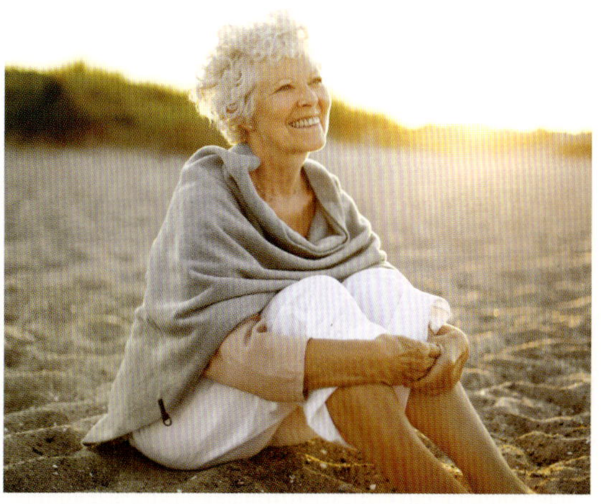

With a slower circulatory system comes poor lymphatic drainage, which is another major contributing factor to unhealthy skin. When lymph drainage is inhibited, an excess of lymph fluid can remain in the tissues, which can create not only stagnation of these waste materials, but also inhibits healthy blood circulation since there is no cellular space to move blood into. This creates systemic backup, which ultimately leaves skin and muscles malnourished and unhealthy.

BENEFITS OF FACE CUPPING

DID YOU KNOW?

While just one face-cupping application yields all of these amazing results, the greatest benefits come with cumulative treatments. They work not only to reduce signs of aging, but also to maintain healthy faces in the future. See *Chapter 8: After a Face-Cupping Treatment* for recommended after-care and treatment plans to reap the greatest benefits from face cupping.

Face cupping provides some incredible benefits to the face. We can see the almost immediate results of cupping here in thermographic images.

Thermographic imaging uses different colors to display the levels of activity in an area. The cooler the coloring is, the less circulation or activity is present in the photographed area. The blue tones indicate lack of circulation, while other colors indicate the progression of temperatures from cold to hot—dark green to green, yellow, orange and red—or the degree of inflammation present in the area. White is the color of most heat (as in the expression "white hot").

In these images, we see the effects of face cupping on our model's face. Naturally, the face is highly vascularized and therefore has a healthy activity of blood circulation before the treatment is applied.

However, once the face-cupping treatment is concluded, we see a dramatic increase in blood circulation across the entire face and neck region. And since the cupping follows the natural lymph drainage routes and contours of the face, we can observe a subtle yet beautiful change in the model's face immediately afterward.

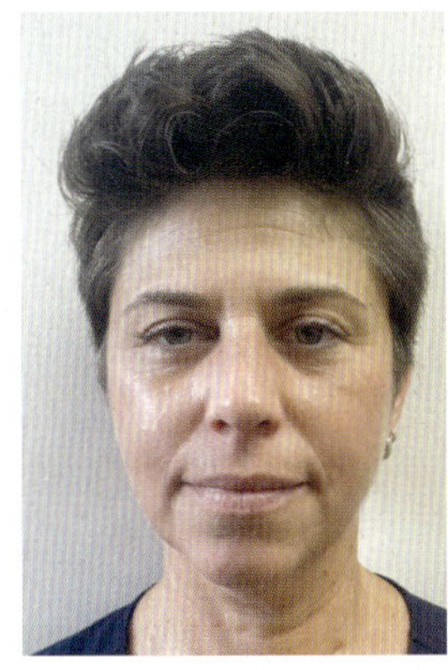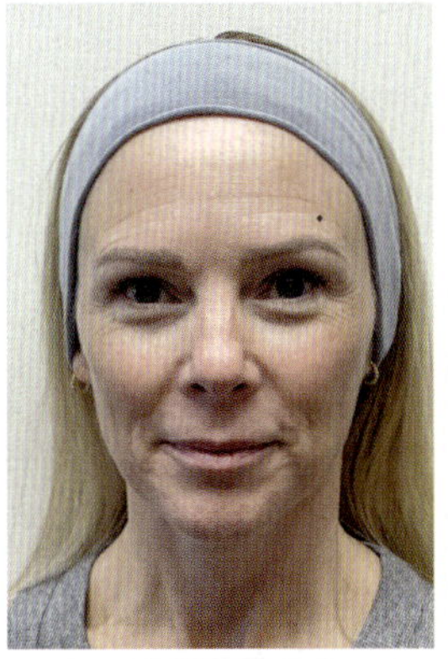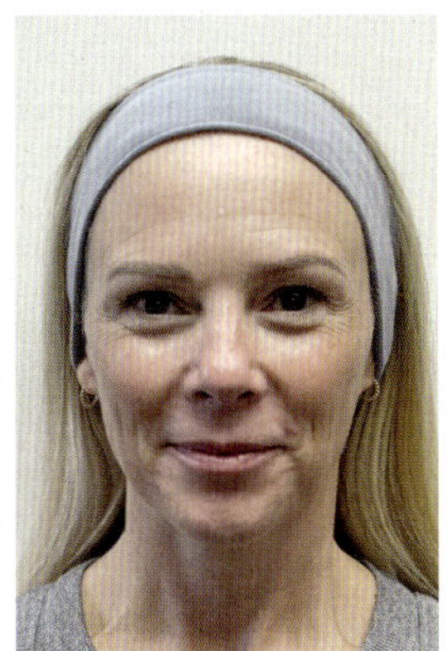

| **BEFORE** | **AFTER 3 TREATMENT** | **BEFORE** | **AFTER 1 TREATMENT** |

Before and after three treatments. Notice more defined face contours and reduced wrinkles. Client reported very relaxed experiences and headache relief at every session.

With beautiful skin, the focus was on forehead wrinkles. In addition to the cosmetic benefits, client reported a wonderfully relaxed sensation and headache relief during and after treatment.

BEFORE

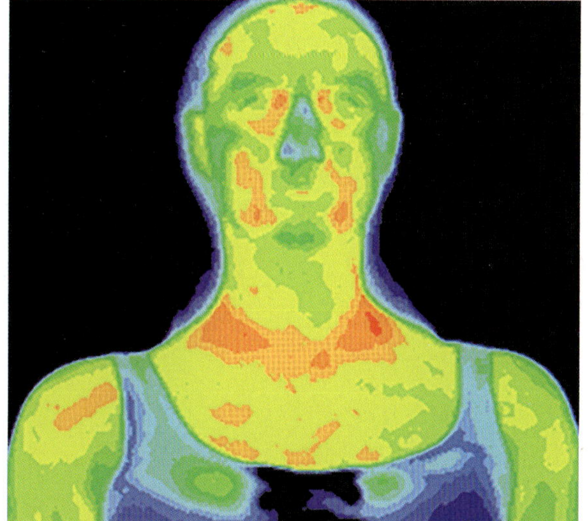 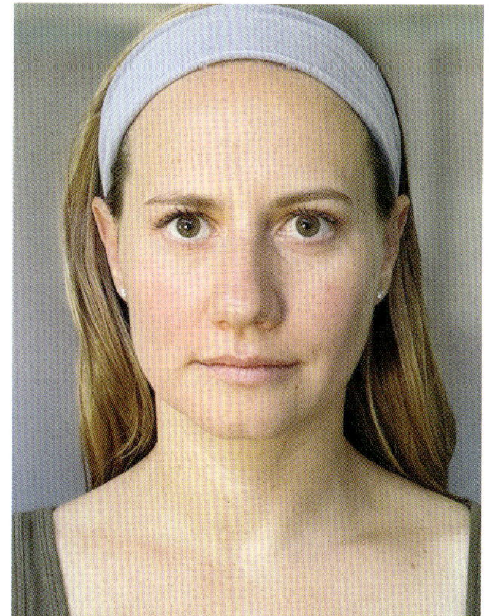

AFTER

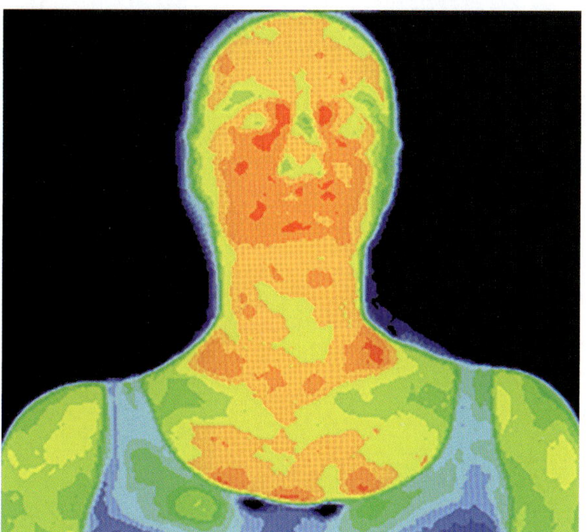 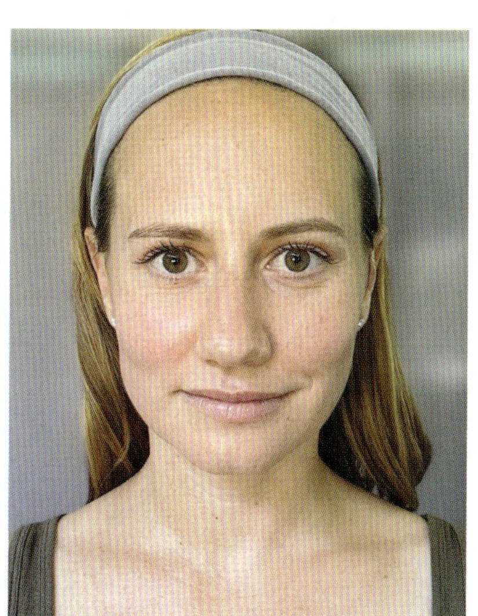

"I loved the facial cupping session and the results were truly amazing! The gentle suction and massage not only relaxed me but also left my skin noticeably smoother and more radiant. I was pleasantly surprised by how refreshed and rejuvenated my face looked afterward. It was such an effective skincare boost!"

—A satisfied client

CHAPTER 7

FACE CUPPING STEP-BY-STEP TREATMENT

OVERVIEW OF TREATMENT PROCESS

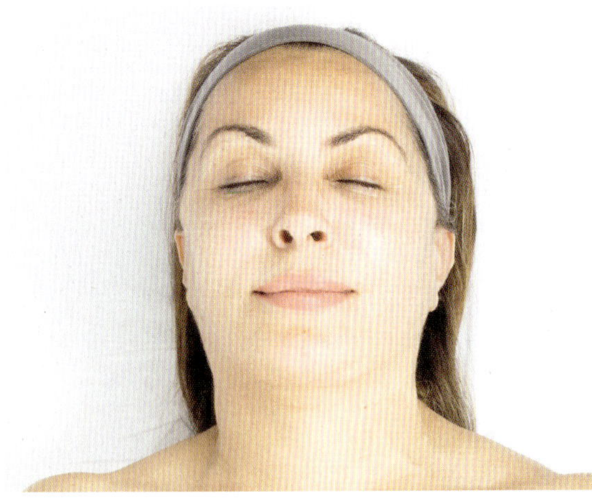

A TOTAL FACE EXPERIENCE

This face-cupping treatment is intended to address the face and head as one unit and in a specific order as it is laid out in this book. Because the treatment generally follows the lymph drainage pathways of the head and neck, each step follows a systematic, logical method of application.

Do not start or work on any region out of order, as this can have an adverse effect on the lymphatic activity in the face and head. Always follow the eight steps laid out here in order.

When done correctly, the treatment simultaneously supports lymph drainage while boosting regional microcirculation. That allows for optimal nutrient-rich distribution and lymph waste removal with every pass of the cup. It also addresses the muscles of the face and any tension they may hold, and helps to alleviate the adhesions between the muscles and skin as they relate to wrinkle formation.

This treatment has multifaceted benefits every time you do it!

WHERE TO BEGIN

When working on both sides of the body, we often work first on one side and then the other. Practitioners usually follow general lymph drainage guidelines and begin with the left side of the body, which houses the more powerful drainage vessels. While working both sides of the face and head simultaneously is the general treatment method of manual lymph drainage, working one side of the face at a time is just as effective and most comfortable for beginners or self-care.

Choosing to start with the left side of the face will stimulate the left thoracic duct, which is responsible for the more powerful drainage in the "terminal" lymph ducts located in the upper chest.

In clinical settings there may be cupping machines that have bifurcated hoses that allow both sides of the face to be treated at the same time. Or perhaps an experienced clinician has two sets of cups and is ambidextrous with their methods of application, which allows them to treat both sides of the face at once.

In this book, however, we will address one side of the face completely, then the other. That means the face-cupping treatment will be demonstrated across the left side of the face. Once the entire left side of the face has been completed, return to *Step 1* and begin treating the right side of the face.

USING THIS BOOK WHILE YOU WORK

The best way to use this book is to work alongside each page you are on, one step at a time. There are step-by-step instructions, including starting points, line(s) of movement, end points and the recommended treatment processes. Also included are wrinkle-reduction options, a lip-plumping option, exceptions, cup-free recommendations, safety point reminders, anatomy tidbits and helpful suggestions wherever applicable.

At the end of the face-cupping step-by-step sequence is a *Face-Cupping Map* (page 158) that lays out the entire treatment process on one page, in one image. This image is useful as a summary, as well as a one-page treatment guide. Once you get familiar with the entire treatment process, you will be able to use this one-page map to follow along with as needed. The charted instructions for each of the eight steps will guide you through the sequence, no page turning necessary.

In general treatment settings, you will be seated at the top of the recipient's head. That is how the images in this book appear, from the practitioner's perspective. If you prefer to position yourself elsewhere (for example, alongside the recipient or standing), please adjust accordingly, keeping the vantage point of this book in mind.

CUP-FREE RECOMMENDATIONS AND EXCEPTIONS

For every step of the treatment process, you will find Cup-Free Options to address exceptions as well as any potential wrinkle-reduction or therapeutic options. Each cup-free recommendation is detailed with directions of application (such as in which direction to create half-circles) intended to replace cup usage with manual lymph drainage techniques wherever necessary. You will find brief notes within each step for any exceptions, but for more detailed information about these items, please review *Chapter 5: Before Beginning Cupping.*

Terms to Know

Proximal means closer to the trunk of core of the body, while **distal** means further from the trunk or core.

Medial means closer to the midline of the body, while **lateral** means further from the midline.

For example, the neck is proximal to the chin, yet distal to the forehead. The mouth is medial to the cheek, while the ear is lateral to it.

FAQ

CAN I FOCUS ON EXTRA CUPPING IN ANY ONE AREA?

A couple of additional lines of movement may add that something extra, for example, in contouring the jawline. You can also consider the Wrinkle-Reduction Options to safely address any focus areas. Nevertheless, if you want to focus on one area, such as the jawline or forehead, be sure to monitor for signs of overworking the skin. You want to avoid cupping marks or swelling. Maintain the average recommended number of passes across the face for an evenly therapeutic and positive face-cupping experience.

PREPARING FOR FACE CUPPING

While not required, a clean face is always ideal for face cupping. Yes, you can work over makeup, but you must apply oil to do the work and that can get messy, not only on the makeup-coated skin but, depending on the makeup, also on the cups. It can become difficult to clean cups when there is makeup on them. Additionally, with a clean face, your pores will be open and skin will be ready for great products to be applied thereafter.

Start with a clean face for the best results.

Note: *Contact lenses do not need to be removed before face-cupping treatment, as the cups should not be in contact with the eye line or eyelid itself.*

Option: If working on newly cleaned skin, consider adding a steam towel or facial steaming, as it will soften the skin, open the pores and serve as great preparation for cupping, allowing the cups to slide across the skin with greater ease.

Now that the skin has been assessed and prepared for the treatment, get the cups, a small hand towel, apply the face oil and get ready to start the face cupping!

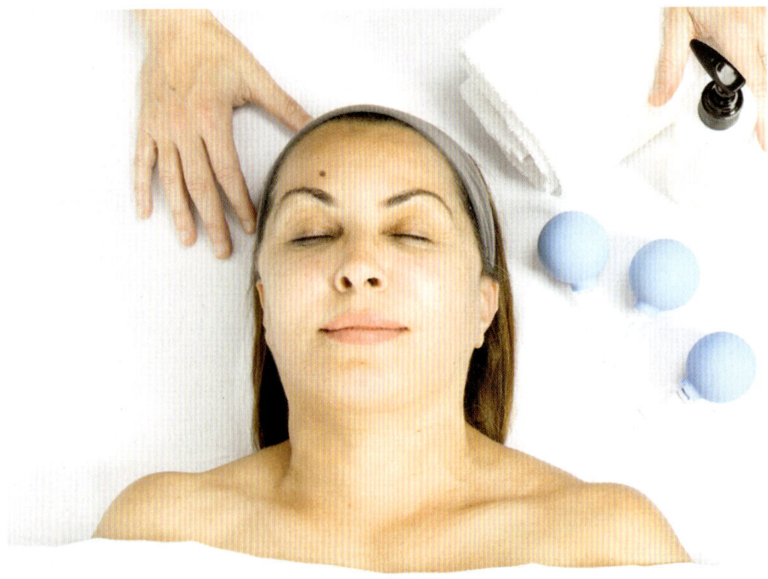

TREATMENT POINTERS

You will want to remember and, if necessary, revisit the following treatment pointers as you work. While each of these points is discussed elsewhere in this book, they are included here for quick reference as you work through the face-cupping treatment process.

- **Use lift-and-release or moving cup techniques—no stationary cups.** There is no need for stationary cups anywhere on the face or neck. (Using stationary cups will likely result in cupping marks!) Use lift-and-release, moving cups or the Morse Code of Cups combination of the two to address every line of movement.
- **Pressure should be light.** In *Chapter 3: How to Use Cups,* we discussed how to use cups most effectively on the face while avoiding the potential for cupping marks. If you want to keep the skin toned and tight—and avoid cupping marks—the suction pressure must be light!
- **Cup should be proportional to the face and larger in size.** Most face-cupping sets only have a few sizes to choose from, but be sure to use the largest cup possible over any given area. For example, you should use a larger cup on the cheek and a smaller cup for the upper lip.
- **Your application should be slow, rhythmic and repetitive.** Work at a slower pace, using rhythmic movements, and apply repetitive passes for the entire application. See page 57 in *Chapter 3* for a full review of the process if needed.
- **Treat the entire face evenly, one cup-width at a time.** Also, to ensure an overall even treatment, repeat each pass three to five times.
- **Follow the step-by-step instructions as written.** It is important to follow the treatment steps as they are described and in the order in which they are written. The very specific step-by-step instructions follow the natural drainage process of the face and head.
- **Use only the lift-and-release technique in the front of the neck—no moving cups.** Remember the no-slide zone in the front of the neck! If you are unsure, do not use cups in the front of the neck. Instead, use your fingertips to do the Cup-Free Options as suggested.

UNDERSTANDING THE UNIVERSAL PASS

Before you begin the face-cupping treatment process, you must be familiar with the front side of the neck, its delicate anatomy and the best method of application for treating this area. Considering how many nerves, blood vessels and lymph vessels are in this part of the neck, you must be aware of a few safety points as you proceed.

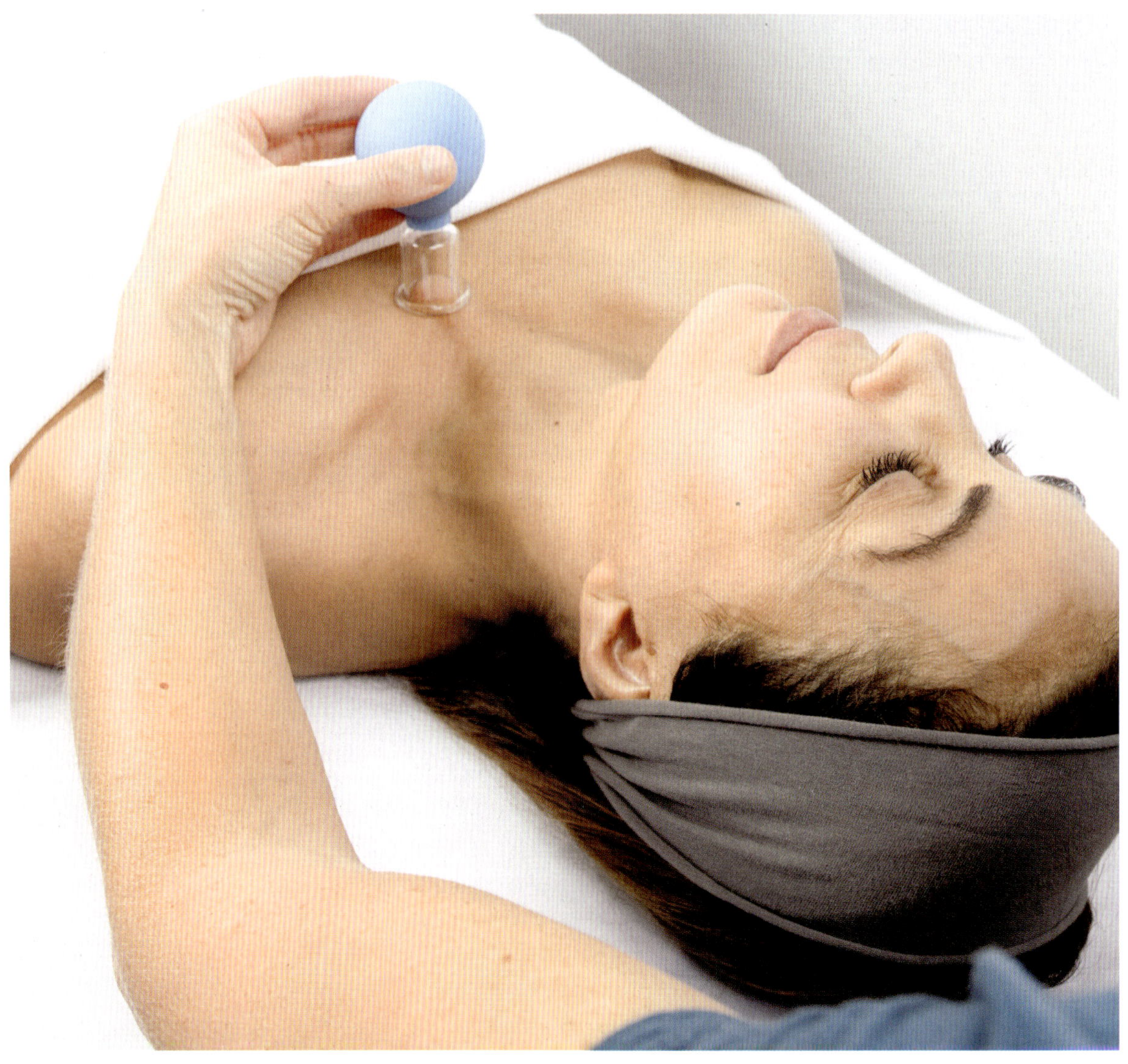

You will begin the treatment with *Step 1: The Upper Chest* and *Step 2: The Front of the Neck,* which focus on the upper chest and neck. The *Universal Pass,* which also focuses on these parts of your body, is a procedure you will be repeating throughout the treatment.

WHY DO THE UNIVERSAL PASS?

Step by step, the cupping treatment in this book follows the general flow of lymph. Think of the Universal Pass as "unclogging a drain" so all the "garbage"—the lymph waste—can be thoroughly and continuously cleared from the region without obstruction.

When you do the Universal Pass after every section has been treated, there will be a clearer path for optimal lymph drainage. Some people can feel fluids collect and move through the front of the neck during the treatment. Others experience an increase in swallowing while working along this drainage route. These are welcome sensations of successful lymph drainage!

WHEN DO YOU DO THE UNIVERSAL PASS?

You will notice that almost every step of the face-cupping treatment in this book ends with the Universal Pass. After every section of the face is cleared, you will find instructions to revisit the Universal Pass, as you want to keep the lymph moving along its disposal route. Be sure that you are comfortable with the process and follow the rules of application every time.

ANATOMY 101

The front of the neck is one of the most vulnerable endangerment sites of the entire body. For more details on this area, review page 64 in *Chapter 4: Safe Cupping Practices.*

Universal Pass Icon

This icon will appear at the end of each step as a reminder to complete the Universal Pass after completing the treatment.

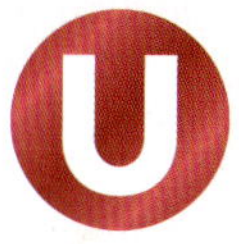

Acknowledging Safety Concerns

While cupping along the front of the neck may seem intimidating, it's not. Every person I have taught how to do this has had immediate success and positive results, as long as they followed the rules. Cupping directly along the SCM muscle is safe since it is a thick muscle, and when manipulating it with a cup you indirectly stimulate all lymph nodes in the region, as these nodes are located close to this powerful neck muscle. There are options to do this with a cup and without.

DID YOU KNOW?

Cupping along the SCM muscle not only stimulates all the lymph drainage; it also offers great relief to neck and jaw tension, too.

WHAT IS THE ROUTE OF THE UNIVERSAL PASS?

The Universal Pass follows the exact same route, or line of movement, that you will address in *Step 1: The Upper Chest* and *Step 2: The Front of the Neck.*

The Universal Pass begins in the soft tissue space at the top of the neck, just below where the ear meets the jaw. We call this area the "jump-off location." (See facing page.)

From there, it travels diagonally down the neck over top of the big neck muscle, the sternocleidomastoid (SCM). You can easily identify the SCM on yourself if you turn your head to the side and bend your head forward slightly; the SCM muscle will "pop" forward for you to identify it. (See photo below.)

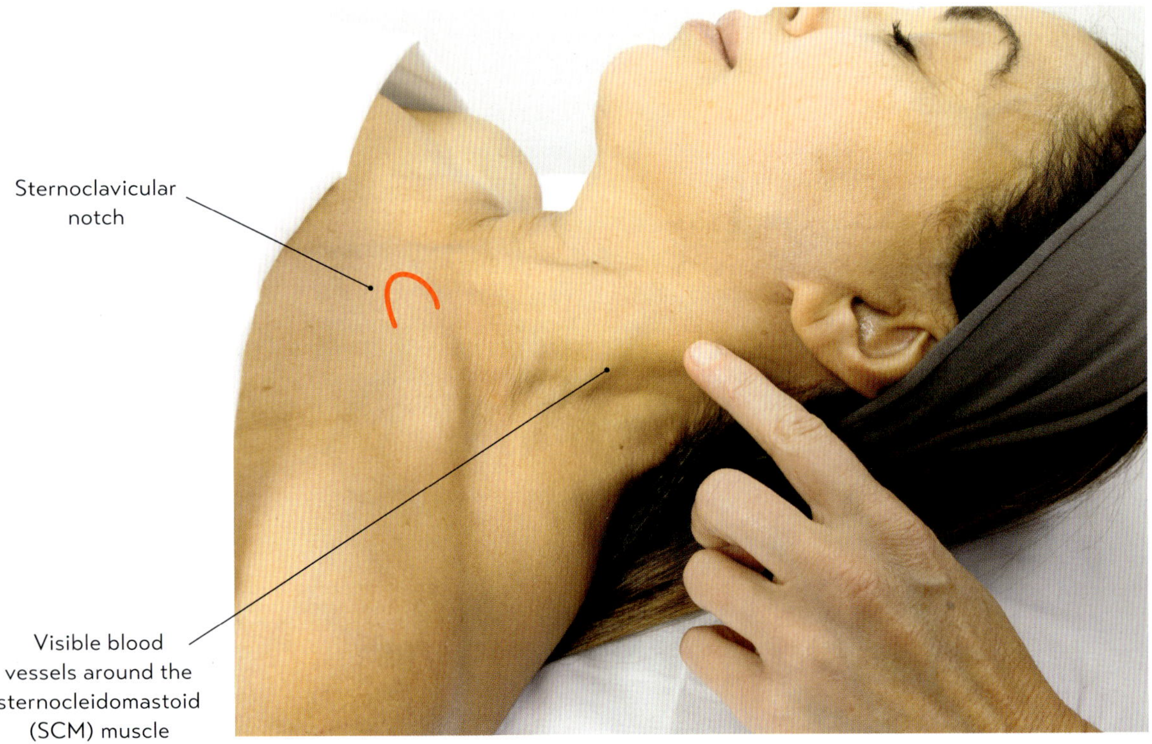

From there, the line of movement proceeds toward the center of the upper chest, travels around the sternoclavicular notch (see photo) and then underneath the collarbones to the center of the upper chest "initial placements," where the entire treatment began.

When you look at the instructional images (pages 112–113), imagine this line of movement as a diagonal *L* for moving *Lymph* fluid.

The Universal Pass

RULES OF APPLICATION FOR THE UNIVERSAL PASS

- **Use only lift-and-release at the front of the neck.** The blood and lymph capillaries that attach just under the skin will be safely stimulated and the nerves will not be irritated. No moving cups or stationary cups here! This region is designated a no-slide zone for safety and optimal effectiveness.
- **Progress in a downward direction only.** As you work, always proceed from the face downward. If you work in an upward direction, you will incorrectly influence the regional lymph fluids, which can potentially lead to head congestion, a headache, or an overload of the lymph nodes.
- **If you come across any visible blood vessels, try to skip over that location entirely.** However, if you happen to attach a cup over these vital blood vessels, especially those that pulse, it should be fine. Just be sure to follow the rules: lift-and-release only in this region. But try to avoid visible blood vessels in the first place.
- **Use slow, rhythmic and repetitive movements.** It is especially important to work mindfully in the front of the neck. Not only is this region hypersensitive, but the vagus nerve travels through the front of the neck. Any erratic, vigorous or aggressive applications in this region could irritate the vagus nerve and cause nausea, dizziness or headaches.

The "Jump-Off" Location

Every time you clear a section of the face and are instructed to follow the Universal Pass, the *jump-off location* mentioned is where the jawline meets the earlobe on the face. This location will be identified again in *Step 3* when you are treating the jawline (see page 124).

Every time you are instructed to do the Universal Pass, you will return to this jump-off location as you leave the face and approach the front of the neck. Once here, be sure to switch to *lift-and-release only* as you revisit the front of the neck.

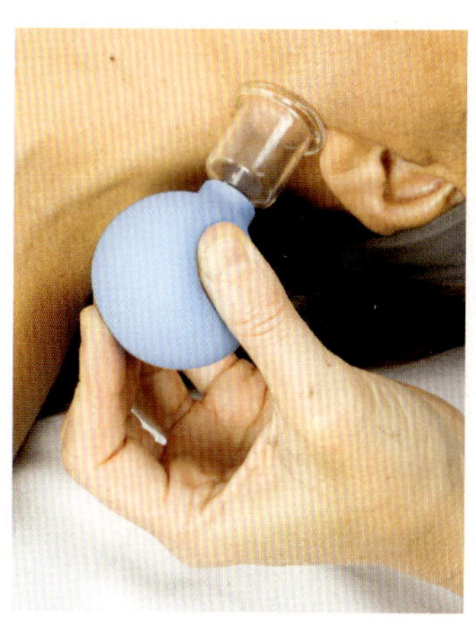

The Universal Pass

LOCATION

This area includes the jump-off location under the earlobe, the front of the neck over the SCM muscle, and the upper chest, just under the collarbone.

STARTING POINT

Start in the soft space of the neck, just under the jump-off location from the face where the jaw meets the earlobe. (See the star in the photo.)

LINE OF MOVEMENT

Follow along down the diagonal *L* line from the starting point, along the SCM muscle, ending at the upper chest locations. (See the Xs.)

END POINT

End at the upper chest, the same upper chest locations addressed in *Step 1*.

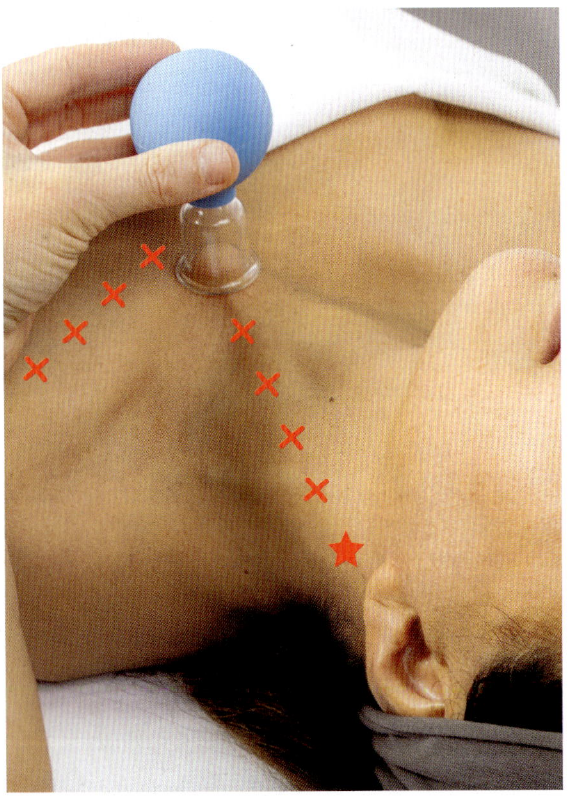

TREATMENT PROCESS

➤ Squeeze the cup, then gently attach it at the starting point.

➤ Simply lift the skin with a little suction, then squeeze the cup again to detach it from the skin's surface. That's the lift-and-release technique!

➤ Repeat this lift-and-release process four or five times down that diagonal line (the Xs) toward the end point in the upper chest (the location of the cup in photo). Think of hopping the cup down the neck as you go.

Once you finish that diagonal *L* line of movement, that's it! This will be the line of movement for every Universal Pass mentioned in the treatment process.

The Universal Pass

CUP-FREE OPTION

If you are unsure about using a cup in this delicate region, simply put the cup down and use this Cup-Free Option. It is simple, safe and incredibly effective.

TREATMENT PROCESS

➤ Use the same starting point, line of movement and end points as instructed with cups, but with your flattened fingertips. Your intention here is only to stretch the skin, to stimulate the underlying lymph capillaries for lymph drainage, so be sure to keep the pressure very light.

➤ Starting at the top of the neck, where the jaw meets the ear, gently use your flattened fingers to contact the skin's surface. Make a half-circle from the top, lightly stretching the skin, forward and down, like an arc of a rainbow. Once you meet the upper chest, the half-circles will go up, over and toward the middle of the collarbone (see photo).

➤ Repeat this gentle skin-stretching, half-circle method of application one hand-width at a time and make your way down to the upper chest area end points. The average neck will accommodate three hand-widths, but everybody is different; what's most important is to address the entire region.

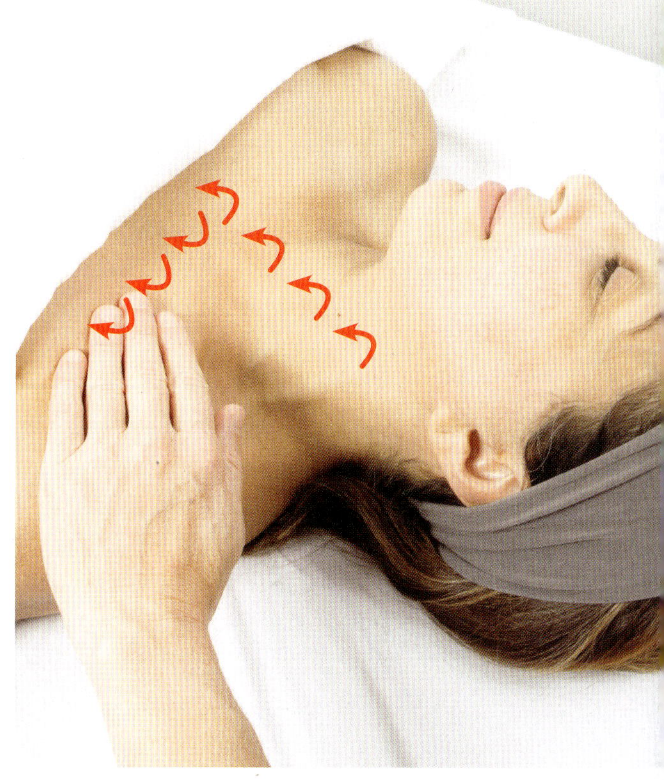

You can use this cup-free method of application any time the Universal Pass is called for in the treatment process.

STEP-BY-STEP FACE CUPPING

The following step-by-step instructions are meant to be followed along with the *Face-Cupping Map* (page 158). The recommended method of treatment is to read each step first, and review it as needed alongside the *Face-Cupping Map*.

To complete the treatment, simply follow the steps, treat each section of the face evenly (three to five passes over every cup-width), repeat the Universal Pass **U** where indicated and then continue to the next step. There are eight steps in all.

Before You Begin

Remember to apply face oil to the entire face before starting face cupping. Be sure to apply a generous amount of recommended oil before you begin. Don't use so much oil that it's dripping, but use more than just a small amount. The average face will allow for a coin-sized amount of oil.

Don't forget to wipe your hands clean after you apply the oil and before you pick up the cup so that it does not slip out of your hands.

The Upper Chest

To begin the process of lymph drainage for the face, we first address the upper chest. Often referred to as the "initial placements," this area is where the entire treatment begins. (It is also the end point for every Universal Pass.) Here is where the lymphatic system is stimulated to promote the drainage process.

WHY CUP THE UPPER CHEST?

Cupping this small area is quick to do and it stimulates all the lymph nodes in the region.

In manual lymph drainage, all lymphatic stimulation begins in this region, addressing the supraclavicular lymph nodes. The exact location to stimulate is located just above the clavicles within the endangerment site of the anterior triangle, so applying the cups in this upper chest space will safely stimulate the lymph nodes indirectly. When this is done correctly, you will see a gentle stretch of the skin above the clavicles, indicating the cup's indirect effect.

Treating this area "unclogs the drain" to clear the path so the lymph collected from the neck and face can drain more efficiently. Every time you travel down the Universal Pass, this is where it will end.

Exceptions

CHEST HAIR?

Follow the Cup-Free Option.

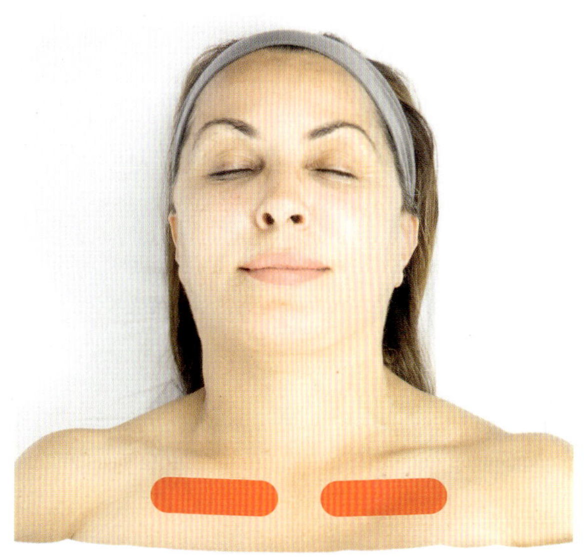

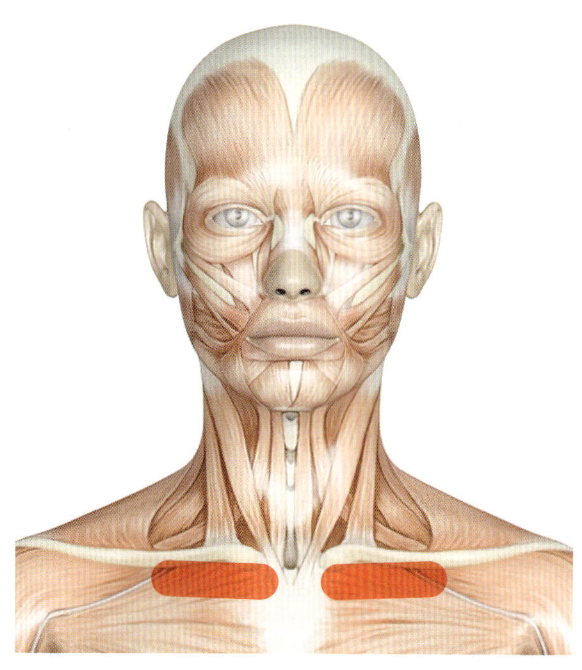

The Upper Chest

LOCATION

This area is just under the clavicle, in the soft tissue space where the clavicle meets the sternum at the sternoclavicular notch, as highlighted in the photo on page 110. The area to address is small: it covers approximately two flattened fingers' width of space, from the sternum to about the middle of the upper chest, directly under the clavicle. The total area covered is three cup placements, 1-2-3.

STARTING POINT

Start directly below the sternoclavicular notch, just off center of the sternum (left or right side, respectively) in the soft tissue space.

LINE OF MOVEMENT

Move from just below the sternoclavicular notch, progressing outward toward the side of the chest.

END POINT

End in the middle of the upper chest, below the center of the clavicle.

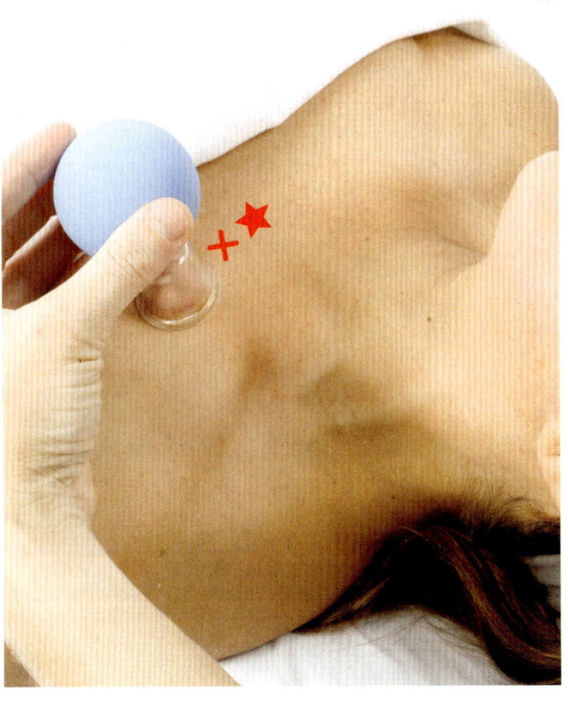

TREATMENT PROCESS

- Attach the cup at the starting point.
- Using lift-and-release, follow this small line of movement across three cup placements. Count them—one, two, three locations.
- That's it. This is a simple, quick and effective way to start the entire drainage process.
- Repeat this line of movement three to five times, then continue to *Step 2: The Front of the Neck*.

The Upper Chest

CUP-FREE OPTION

If a cup will not attach to the skin in this section for any reason (for example, chest hair, clothing) or if you have reason to prefer not to use a cup in this area, follow the Cup-Free Option and use your fingers instead to gently stimulate the lymph drainage pathways.

TREATMENT PROCESS

Using the same starting point, line of movement and end points as instructed with cups, use your flattened fingertips to create small half-circles across the surface of the skin.

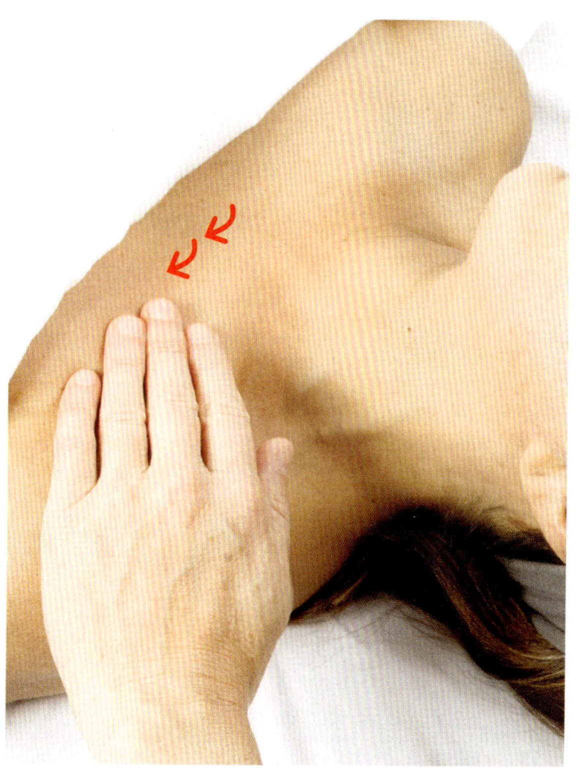

➤ As you treat the left side of the upper chest, use your left hand (as in photo); if you are working on the right side of the upper chest, use your right hand.

➤ Starting at the midline and progressing outward, gently use your flattened fingers to contact the skin's surface and make a half-circle, lightly stretching the skin up, forward and down (see photo), like the arc of a rainbow.

➤ Completely remove your fingertips from the skin after every half-circle is completed, then "step" your fingertips to the next location and repeat the process.

➤ Repeat these gentle, skin-stretching half-circles one finger-tipped placement at a time to address these upper chest points. The average person's upper chest region will accommodate three hand placements.

➤ Repeat this line of movement three to five times, then continue to *Step 2: The Front of the Neck.*

The Front of the Neck

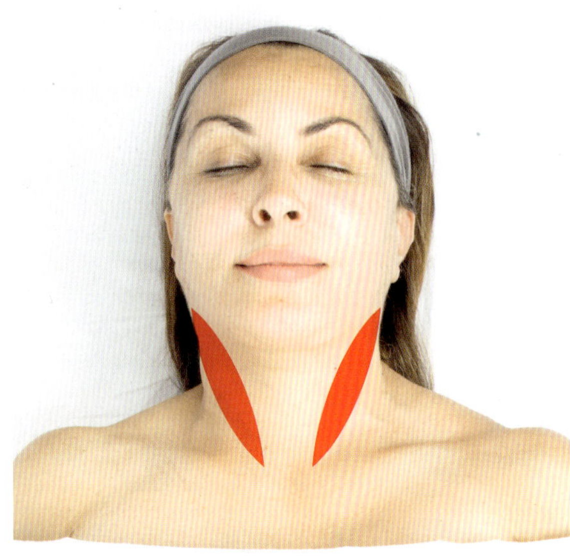

When stimulating lymph drainage for the face, it is important to address the neck. The front of the neck contains many lymph nodes that collectively drain the face and head, as well as muscles that contribute to tension throughout the face, jaw and neck. However, since this location also contains delicate endangerment sites that make it one of the most vulnerable parts of the body, we must proceed with caution. For more information about this endangerment site, see page 67 in *Chapter 4: Safe Cupping Practices.*

WHY CUP THE FRONT OF THE NECK?

Cupping along the front of the neck is a very important part of this face-cupping treatment. Working along this line of movement will safely stimulate the many lymph nodes located here, initiating lymph drainage for the entire neck, face and head. Cupping through this area also helps to release tension in some potentially tight neck muscles, especially the strong SCM muscle, and that release provides relief to both the neck and jaw.

CUP PLACEMENT AND SAFELY CUPPING THE FRONT OF THE NECK

For this step, you will apply lift-and-release along the sternocleidomastoid or SCM muscle several times. You will generally make six to nine passes along this muscle during this step, throughly stimulating lymph drainage.

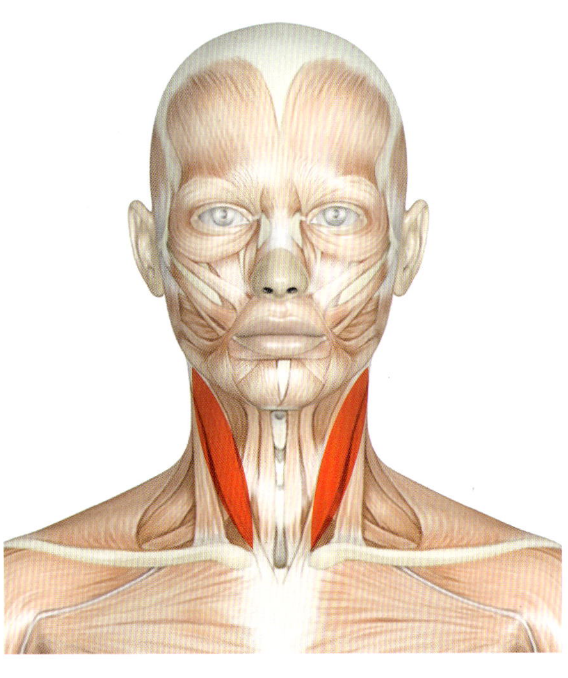

Also, you will generally cover this line of movement with several cup placements. By "generally," I mean that cup placements are not edge-to-edge along this line of movement. Instead, you "hop" the cup along the SCM muscle with every pass. If you were to draw a line, cup placements would resemble evenly spaced polka dots, and not a string of pearls, along the SCM muscle.

A wider or longer neck will have more placements (four to six), while a thinner or shorter neck will have fewer placements (three to five).

THE SAFEST LINES OF MOVEMENT

While following the SCM muscle, be sure to observe for any obvious blood vessels, as some people may have more prominent blood vessels than others. Work mindfully and avoid any visible blood vessels. Skipping over any obvious vasculature and working through this region in a relaxed manner is the best method of application for the blood vessels, lymph nodes and nerves located here. (See the illustration on page 110.)

SAFETY REMINDER

Remember that lift-and-release is the only technique to be used in the front of the neck. Be sure also to use slower, rhythmic methods of application as you work down the neck. Any vigorous or fast-paced cupping here could irritate the many nerves here, including the vagus nerve.

Exceptions

FACIAL HAIR?

Follow the Cup-Free Option.

TURN THE HEAD FOR THIS STEP

Turn your client's head to the right for this step and to the left when treating the right side of the face. This allows for better visibility of blood vessels and creates greater space for ease of application. If the client is uncomfortable with their head turned (because of a stiff neck, for example), you will want to observe the side of the neck closely as you work.

This is not required for every treatment, but it is a good method of application as you familiarize yourself with cupping through the front of the neck. Once this step is finished, your client's head can turn forward again for the rest of the treatment.

The Front of the Neck

LOCATION

This area includes the jump-off location under the earlobe and the front of the neck over the SCM muscle, as with the Universal Pass.

STARTING POINT

Start in the soft space of your neck, just below the jump-off location where the jaw meets the earlobe. (See the star in the photo.) With three possible lines of movement, the starting point will always be the same.

LINE OF MOVEMENT

Picture this line of movement as a diagonal *L* for moving *Lymph*. Follow along down the diagonal *L* line from the starting point, along the SCM muscle, under the collarbones, ending at the upper chest locations. (See the Xs.) This line follows your SCM muscle (highlighted in photo on page 110) and is exactly the same as in the Universal Pass.

END POINT

End below the middle of the clavicle, in the upper chest locations.

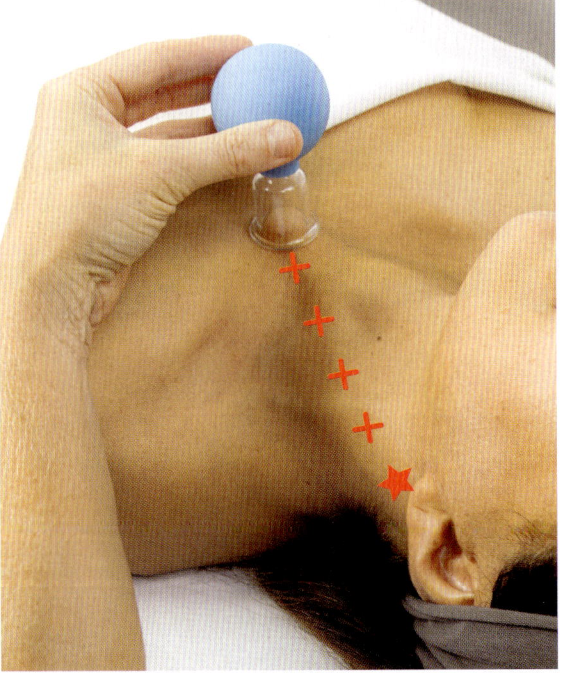

TREATMENT PROCESS

➤ Attach the cup at the starting point.
➤ Using lift-and-release only, follow the line of movement down the side of the neck, along the SCM muscle and into those upper chest, initial placement locations.
➤ Repeat this lift-and-release treatment process along the line of movement three to five times.
➤ Continue to *Step 3: The Jawline.*

The Front of the Neck

CUP-FREE OPTION

If cups will not work for whatever reason in this region (for example, facial hair, vascular issues), or if you prefer not to use a cup in this area, use your fingertips to follow this Cup-Free Option to gently follow the lymph drainage pathways.

TREATMENT PROCESS

Using the same starting point, line of movement and end point as instructed with cups, use your flattened fingertips to create small half-circles across the surface of the skin.

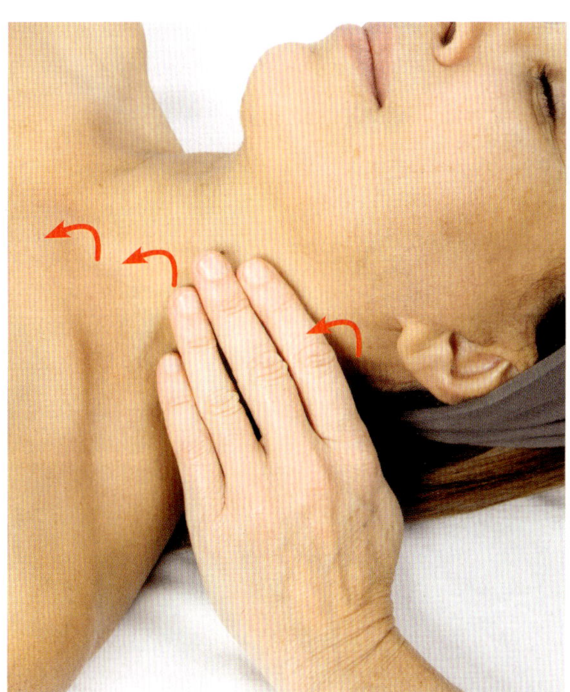

- Use the same hand as the side of the neck you are treating for this Cup-Free Option. When you are working on the left side of the face, use your left hand (as in the photo), and when you are working on the right side of the face, use your right hand.
- Begin your fingertip half-circles at the top of the neck in the soft tissue space just below where the jaw meets the ear.
- Starting at the top of neck, gently use your flattened fingers to contact the skin's surface and make a half-circle, lightly stretching the skin forward and down (see photo), like an arc of a rainbow.
- Completely remove your fingertips from the skin after every half-circle is completed, then "step" your fingertips to the next placement and repeat.
- Repeat these gentle skin-stretching, half-circles one hand-width at a time and make your way down to the upper chest area end points. The average neck will accommodate three or four hand-widths.
- Repeat this line of movement six to nine times.
- Continue to *Step 3: The Jawline.*

The Jawline

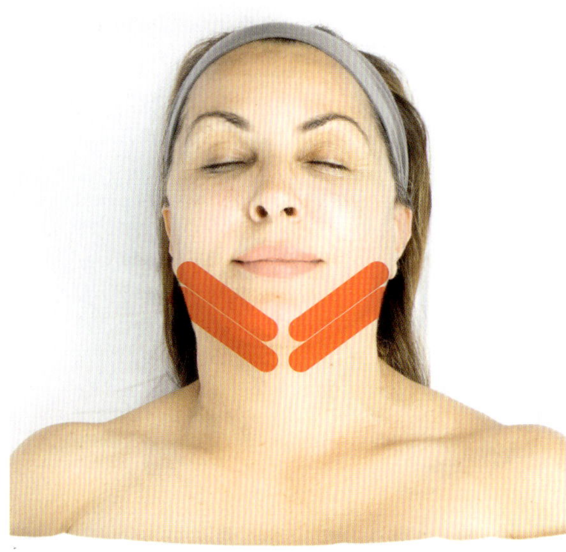

The jawline is a location where the skin can begin to sag, creating those concentrated areas of loosened skin referred to as jowls. Additionally, this area has many blood vessels, lymph nodes and muscles, so any tension can not only inhibit optimal circulation to the skin, but also potentially contribute to muscle pains in the jaw and general neck region.

WHY CUP ALONG THE JAWLINE?

Cupping along the jawline helps to improve tone, appearance and the general health of the face. As there are many lymph nodes and muscles located here, cupping along the jawline is incredibly therapeutic for the overall lymphatic activity of the face and head. Moreover, as you move a cup along here, you may encounter "speed bumps" and restrictions associated with TMJD and jaw tension. Cupping along the jawline can offer relief to some of these jaw and neck muscles, too.

For the greatest benefits, we divide the jawline into two parts: *Below the Jawline* and *Above the Jawline*. Note that there are Cup-Free Options for both parts.

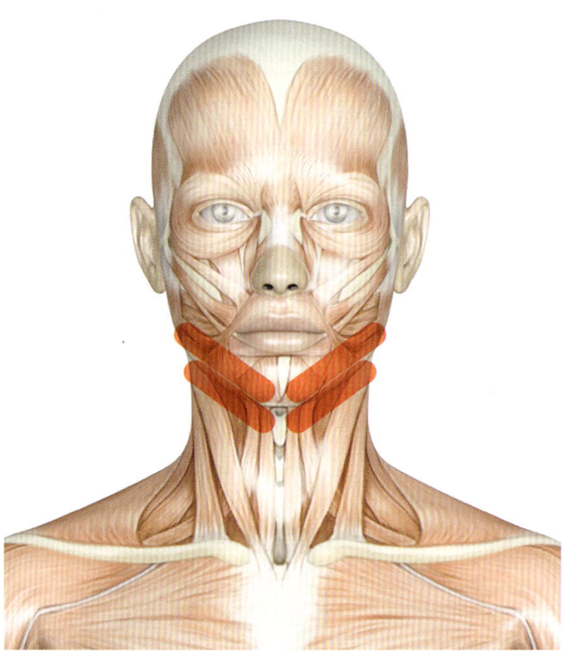

LYMPHATICS 101

Many people are familiar with the lymphatic activity here, as several lymph nodes located along the underside of the jawline are the first to swell when we notice head congestion or the onset of any cold or flu-like illness.

Exceptions

FACIAL HAIR?

Option 1: For shorter or thinner facial hair, follow the Cup-Free Option.

Option 2: For longer or thicker facial hair, gently pinch and lightly pull the facial hair as you travel along the line of movement.

ACNE?

Option 1: Follow the Cup-Free Option.

Option 2: Use lift-and-release as you encounter acne; moving cups are not recommended over areas containing pimples and acne blemishes that could potentially "pop." If any blemishes should pop, cease working over that area for the remainder of the treatment.

JAW TENSION?

If you encounter a tension-related "speed bump" along the way, do not force the cup to move across it. Instead, revert to the lift-and-release technique to get across that section. Then finish that line of movement with lift-and-release, moving cups or a combination of the two using the Morse Code of Cups. Interested in more therapeutic options for TMJD? See page 81 in *Chapter 5: Before Beginning Cupping.*

VERY LOOSE SKIN?

Option 1: Use lift-and-release to address this line of movement. With time, as tonicity improves, moving cups will be possible.

Option 2: Use one hand to manage the cup and the other hand to hold the skin taut. This two-handed method of application anchors the loose skin as you move the cup along the line of movement and it is meant to be gentle and supportive.

For more details about any exceptions, review pages 78–84 in *Chapter 5: Before Beginning Cupping.*

Below the Jawline

LOCATION

This area includes the underside of the face and jawbone, and does not cross the front of the neck and throat, which contains endangerment sites (see page 67).

STARTING POINT

Start in the center of the jawline, under the chin.

LINE OF MOVEMENT

Follow along the underside of the entire jawbone, moving toward the ear.

END POINT

End in front of the ear and under the jawbone where the jaw meets the ear. (See cup location in photo.) This is just below the jump-off location, where the Universal Pass begins.

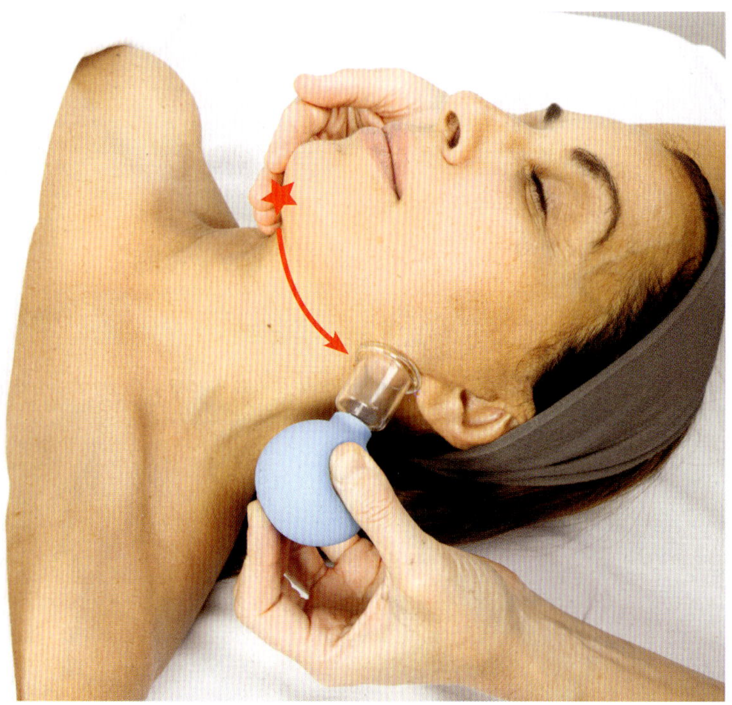

TREATMENT PROCESS

➤ Attach the cup at the starting point and follow the line of movement using lift-and-release and/or moving cups to the end point.

➤ Repeat this line of movement three to five times.

➤ Repeat the Universal Pass **U** one to three times before proceeding.

➤ Continue to the next part of *Step 3, Above the Jawline.*

THE "JUMP-OFF" LOCATION

See page 111 for a photo and more information on the jump-off location. The end points for the *Step 3: The Jawline* treatments are at or near the jump-off location.

Below the Jawline

CUP-FREE OPTION

If the cups will not work for whatever reason in this region (facial hair, cosmetic implants, etc.), or if you prefer not to use a cup in this area, use your fingertips to follow this Cup-Free Option to gently follow the lymph drainage pathways.

TREATMENT PROCESS

Using the same starting point, line of movement and end point as instructed with cups, use your flattened fingertips to create small half-circles across the surface of the skin.

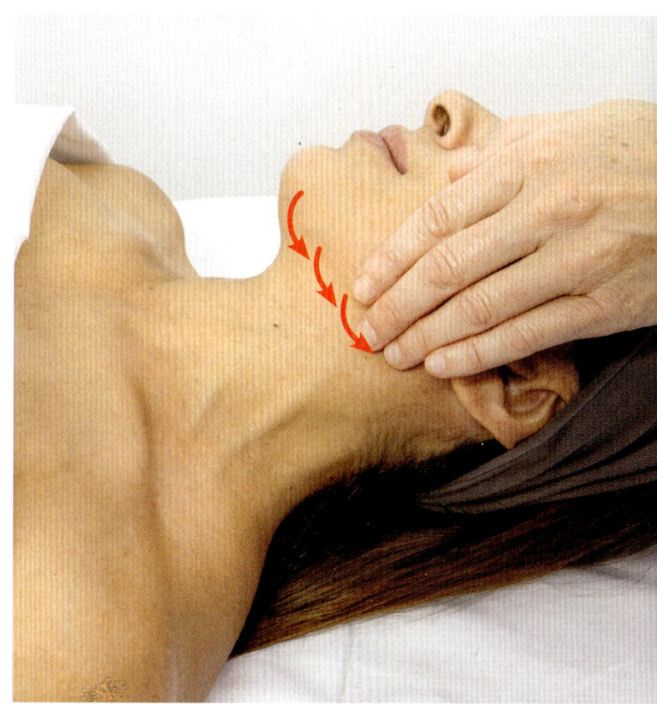

- ➤ Use the same hand as the side of the neck you are treating for this Cup-Free Option. When you are working on the left side of the face, use your left hand and progress toward the left ear (as in the photo), and when you are working on the right side of the face, use your right hand and progress toward the right ear.
- ➤ Begin your fingertip half-circles in the center of the jawline, under the chin.
- ➤ Starting at the midline, gently use your flattened fingers to lightly stretch this skin in a half-circle down and around, toward the ear.
- ➤ Completely remove your fingertips from the skin after every half-circle is completed, then "step" your fingertips to the next placement and repeat.
- ➤ Repeat these half-circles one hand-width at a time to address the underside of the jawline. The average person's lower jawline will accommodate three or four hand placements.
- ➤ Repeat this line of movement three to five times.
- ➤ Repeat the Universal Pass 🅤 one to three times before proceeding.
- ➤ Continue to the next part of *Step 3: Above the Jawline.*

Above the Jawline

LOCATION
This area is below the mouth and along the jawbone and ends in front of the earlobe. Be sure to not pull any lip tissue into the cup, as that is not part of this section.

STARTING POINT
Start in the center of the chin, under the lower lip.

LINE OF MOVEMENT
Follow along the entire jawbone, progressing toward the ear.

END POINT
End in front of the earlobe, where the jawbone meets the ear. (See the cup location in photo.) This is also the jump-off location, where the Universal Pass begins.

TREATMENT PROCESS
➤ Attach the cup at the starting point.
➤ Follow the line of movement using lift-and-release and/or moving cups to the end point.
➤ Repeat this line of movement three to five times.
➤ Repeat the Universal Pass **U** one to three times before proceeding to *Step 4: The Mouth Area*.

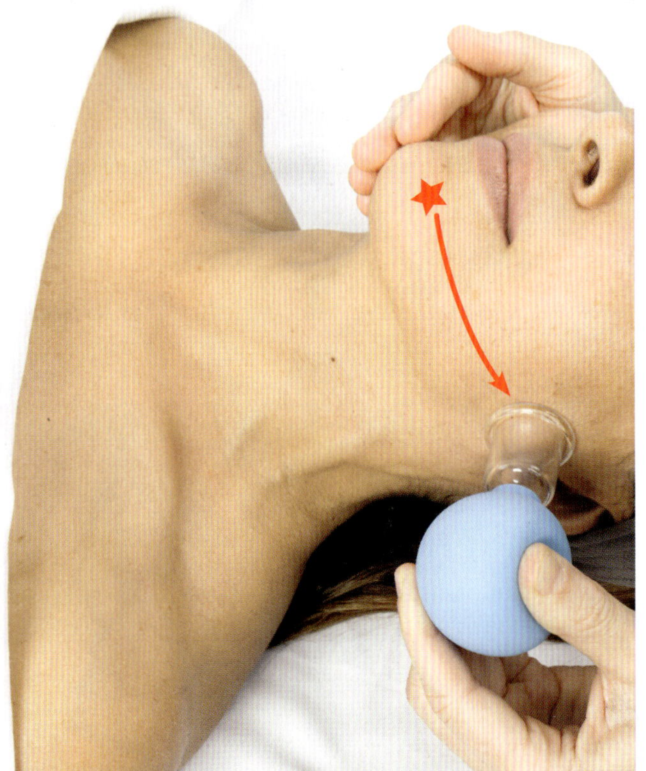

Above the Jawline

CUP-FREE OPTION

If the cups will not work for whatever reason in this region (facial hair, very loose skin, etc.), or if you prefer not to use a cup in this area, use your fingertips to follow this Cup-Free Option to gently follow the lymph drainage pathways.

TREATMENT PROCESS

Using the same starting point, line of movement and end point as instructed with cups, use your flattened fingertips to create small half-circles across the surface of the skin.

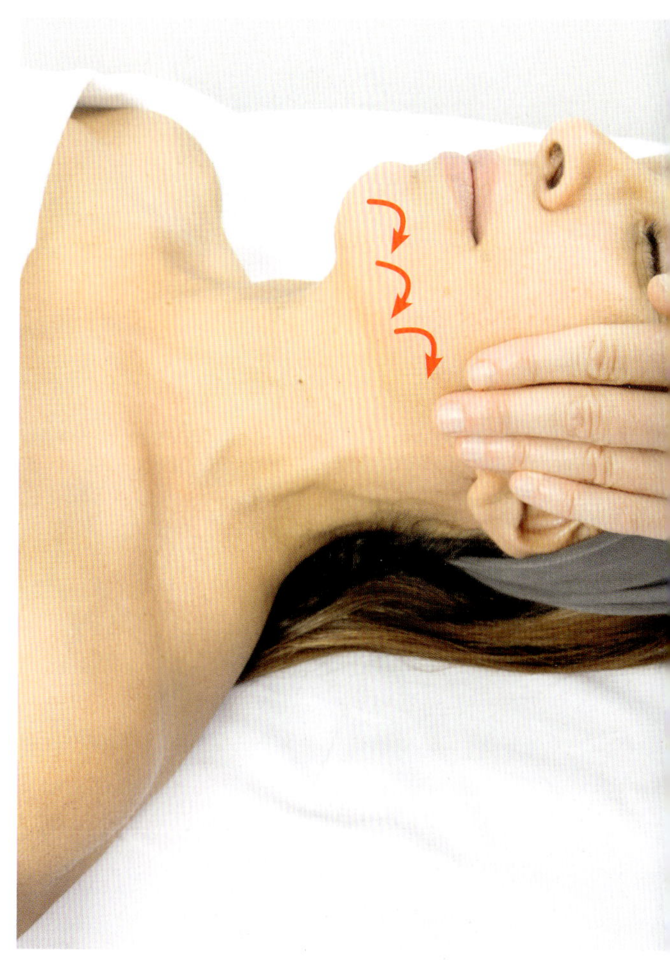

➤ Use the same hand as the side of the face you are treating for this Cup-Free Option. When you are working on the left side of the face, use your left hand and progress toward the left ear (as in the photo): if you are working on the right side of the face, use your right hand and progress toward the right ear.

➤ Begin your fingertip half-circles in the center of the chin, below the lower lip.

➤ Starting at the midline, gently use your flattened fingers to contact the skin's surface and make a half-circle, lightly stretching the skin up and around toward the ear.

➤ Completely remove your fingertips from skin after every half-circle is completed, then "step" your fingertips to the next placement and repeat.

➤ Repeat these gentle, skin-stretching half-circles one hand-width at a time to address the area along the upper jawline. The average person's upper jawline will accommodate three or four hand placements.

➤ Repeat this line of movement three to five times.

➤ Repeat the Universal Pass **U** one to three times before proceeding to *Step 4: The Mouth Area.*

The Mouth Area

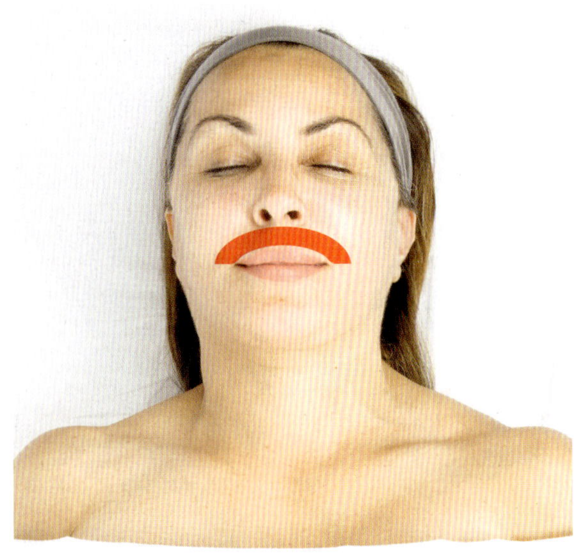

This is a very small region to address, so it will not take much time to do. Some people have very tight lip muscles and prominent wrinkles that require more attention, but for most, this is a quick and easy step. People who have facial hair may also require an exceptional treatment process as described below.

The line of movement is short; it ends at the side of the mouth, where *Step 5: The Cheeks* begins. (Be sure to attach the cup to the skin of the face, and not to the lip tissue itself.)

While this step works on the area directly above the mouth, there is also a Lip-Plumping Option if there is interest in directly treating the lips. (See page 131.)

WHY CUP THE MOUTH AREA?

Cupping in the mouth area can improve the appearance of the skin there; in particular, treating the muscles that surround the mouth can provide relief from the small wrinkles lines that occur here. And even though there are no lymph nodes located directly around the mouth, cupping this small area will help move lymph from this region and into lymph nodes located nearby in the cheek and jawline areas.

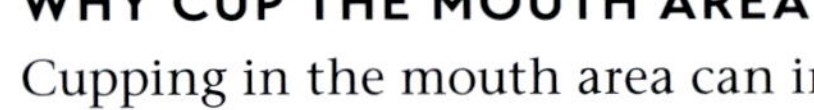

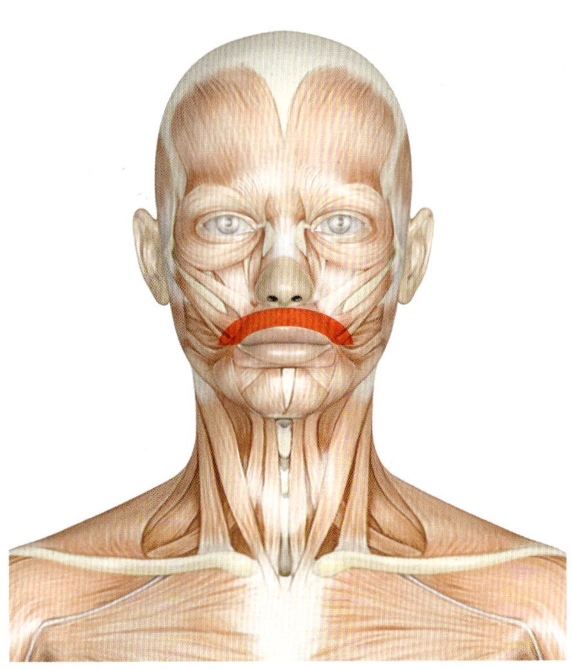

Exceptions

FACIAL HAIR?

Option 1: For shorter or thinner facial hair, follow the Cup-Free Option.

Option 2: For longer or thicker facial hair, gently pinch and lightly pull the facial hair as you follow the line of movement.

The Mouth Area

LOCATION

You are working directly above the upper lip; be sure to attach the cup to the skin, not the lip tissue or the nostril.

STARTING POINT

Start directly above the center of the upper lip, under the nose.

LINE OF MOVEMENT

Move along the upper lip to the side of the mouth; this is a very short distance.

END POINT

End at the edge of the mouth. This is approximately where the nasolabial wrinkles would form.

Note: *Be sure to use a smaller cup as you begin to treat the mouth area.*

TREATMENT PROCESS

➤ Attach the cup at the starting point.
➤ Follow this small line of movement to the end point using lift-and-release and/or moving cups.
➤ Repeat this line of movement three to five times.
➤ There is no need to do the Universal Pass after treating this small area. Once this section is completed, continue to *Step 5: The Cheeks*.

If interested, proceed to the *Lip-Plumping Option* now, before continuing to *Step 5*. Or you can can do this option at the very end of the entire treatment. See page 131.

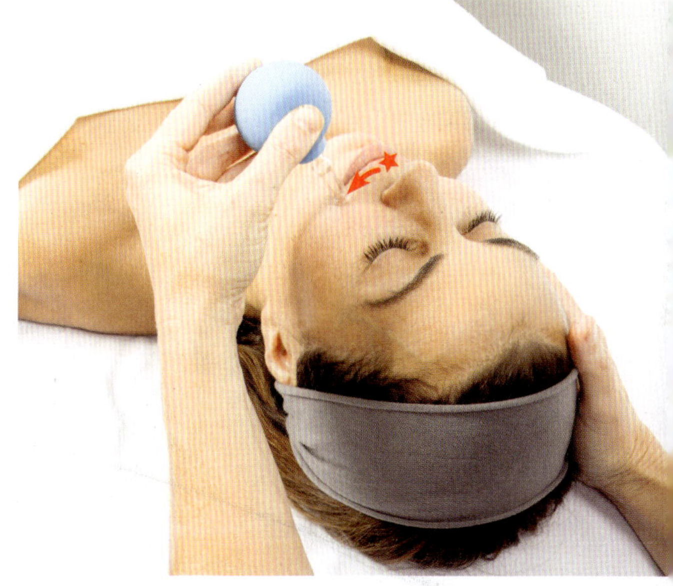

The Mouth Area

CUP-FREE OPTION

If the cup will not attach to the skin in this area for any reason (facial hair, cosmetic injections, etc.), use your fingertips to follow this Cup-Free Option to gently follow the lymph drainage pathways.

Using the same starting point, line of movement and end point as instructed with cups, use your flattened fingertips to create small half-circles across the surface of the skin. Remember, do not include the lip tissue in this treatment, only the skin above the mouth.

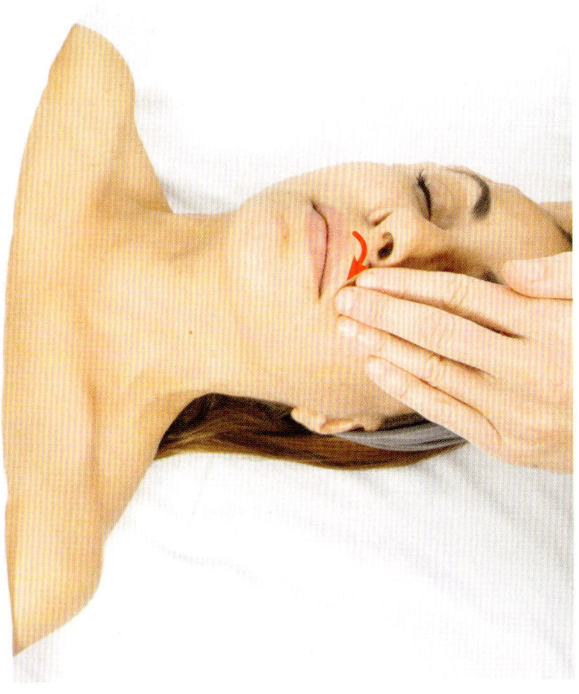

TREATMENT PROCESS

➤ Use the same hand as the side of the face you are treating for this Cup-Free Option. When you are working on the left side of the face, use your left hand and progress toward the left side of the mouth (as in the photo); when you are working on the right side of the face, use your right hand and progress toward the right side of the mouth.

➤ Use your fingertips to make small half-circles, lightly stretching the surface of the skin. The half-circles travel upward and around toward the cheek (left or right respectively).

➤ Use this gentle skin-stretching, half-circle method of application to cover the upper lip region entirely. This is a very small area, so you will make only a few placements here.

➤ Repeat this line of movement three to five times.

➤ There is no need to do the Universal Pass after treating this small area. Once this section is completed, continue to *Step 5: The Cheeks*.

The Mouth Area

LIP-PLUMPING OPTION

As with all cupping applications, the lip tissue responds to cups and the stimulation of circulation, which in turn stimulates collagen production when treated. If you want to add this application in a clinical practice, I highly recommend you use glass cups for sterilization purposes since the cup goes directly on top of the lips. The cup size should be large enough to encompass both upper and lower lips together, but not too large, since you need to make a few cup placements across the mouth for best results. If cupping for self-care, silicone cups are fine.

If you choose to add this option to the treatment, you should do so when you are addressing the mouth area, after *Step 4* has been completed. You should treat the entire mouth all at once, but whether you choose to do this option after *Step 4* is complete on the left or right side is up to you. Or you could do this option at the very end of the entire treatment, since drool may be extracted. (See note, right.)

Note: *The possibility of saliva and drool being sucked into the cups is very strong. As this is a typical response to cupping the lips, wash your cups thoroughly after use. You do not have to wash the cup immediately, but you should wipe the fluids from the cup before proceeding with the rest of the treatment.*

TREATMENT PROCESS

➤ Beginning at the midline of the mouth and progressing toward the side of the mouth (left or right), apply a larger cup directly over the mouth area using lift-and-release only. Be sure to cover both upper and lower lips at the same time.

➤ Repeat this line of movement five to ten times, depending on how much "plumping" is desired. A little goes a long way, so do not to overdo it. Ten passes (on each side) is plenty for each treatment.

➤ Once this step is completed, continue to *Step 5: The Cheeks.*

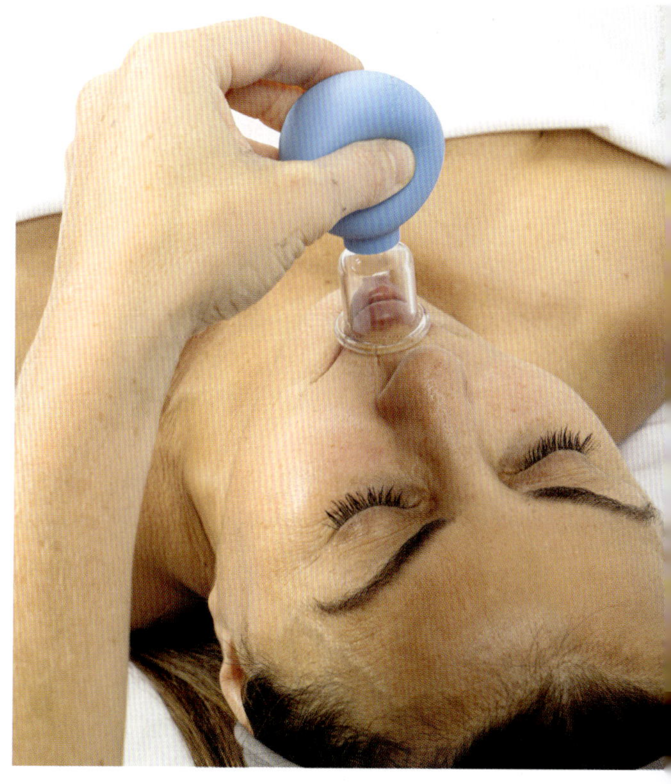

The Cheeks

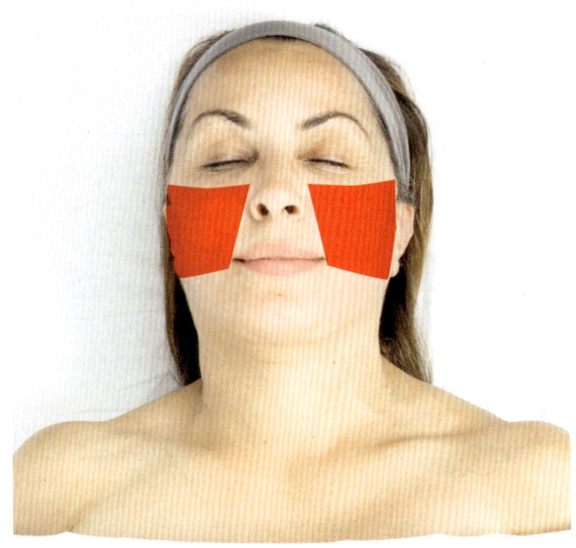

The cheeks cover a large area of the face, showcasing our skin, healthy or otherwise. The cheeks also house the paranasal sinuses, alongside the nose, which are often involved with sinus congestion.

Moreover, the cheeks cover a lot of important musculature, including the many muscles used in smiling and laughing, and the often-tight muscles in the jaw region. As already mentioned, the temporomandibular joint of the jaw—the TMJ area—is a common location of tension. Tension here can also contribute to wrinkles and distorted skin textures across the face.

WHY CUP THE CHEEKS?

Cupping across the cheeks greatly improves circulation in the face, which contributes to that healthy glow that face cupping is famous for. Cupping across this area will also allow for much-needed muscle relaxation, which benefits not only wrinkles but the tension associated with the entire jaw area.

Note that there is also a Wrinkle-Reduction Option for this step.

CHEEK SIZE AND CUP CHOICE

Be sure to use a larger cup size here, as a smaller cup across this larger area could result in cupping marks. Using smaller cups over such a large, vascularized area creates focused suction, which is not what you want to provide here.

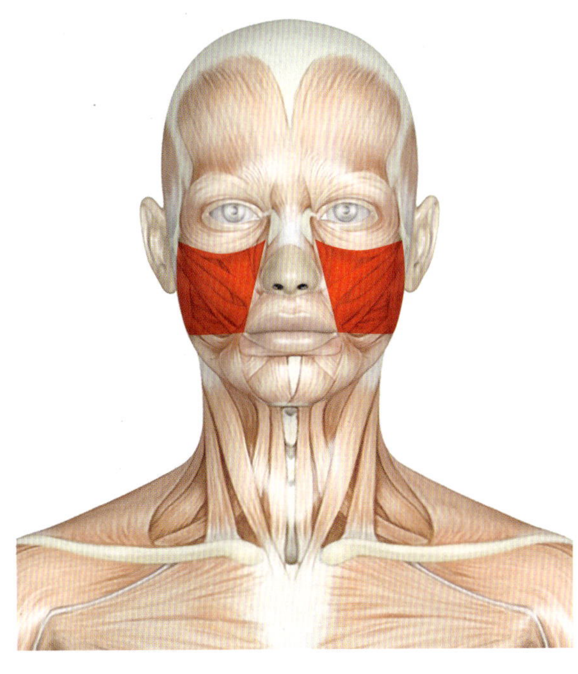

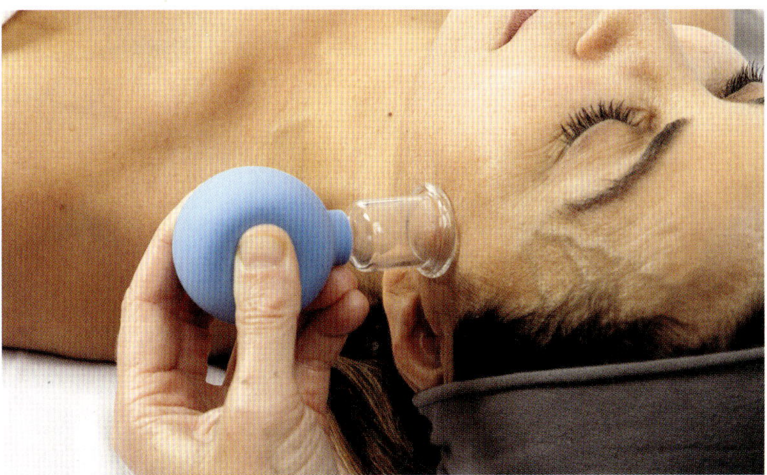

Cupping over TMJ area

Also, because everyone has different anatomical features, measure the cheek area for each individual person according to the borders described in the location note for the treatment process (on page 134). While the average adult cheek area fits two larger cup-widths, a longer face may fit three cup-widths to cover the entire cheek area. No matter what the size, the cheek area ends when the top edge of the cup is close to the delicate eye tissue region. That area is separately addressed in *Step 7: The Eyes*.

What About Cupping the Nose?

When doing face cupping, the primary goal is to influence lymph drainage, regional blood flow and muscle tension. Many steps in this treatment will affect the nose indirectly, so there is no need to treat it directly. However, should you choose to use a very small cup on the sides of the nose or directly on top of it, I recommend you do so during this step, *Step 5: The Cheeks*. You can work on the sides of the nose as you treat the topmost line of the cheek, since it flows into that line of movement naturally.

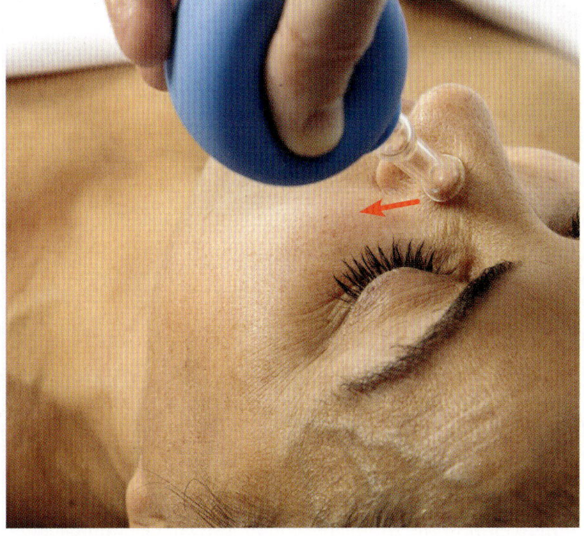

Exceptions

FACIAL HAIR?

If cupping over the facial hair is unavailable, there are two options here.

Option 1: For shorter or thinner facial hair, follow the Cup-Free Option.

Option 2: For longer or thicker facial hair, gently pinch and lightly pull the facial hair as you travel along the line of movement.

ACNE?

Option 1: Follow the Cup-Free Option.

Option 2: Use the lift-and-release as you encounter any acne; moving cups are not recommended. If any blemishes should "pop," cease working over that area for the remainder of the treatment.

JAW TENSION?

If you encounter a tension-related "speed bump" along the way, do not force the cup to move across it. Instead, revert to lift-and-release to get across that section. Then finish that line of movement with lift-and-release, moving cups or a combination of the two using the Morse Code of Cups. Interested in more therapeutic options for TMJD? See page 82 in *Chapter 5*.

RECENT INJECTIONS?

After thirty days post-injection, there are two options:

Option 1: Follow the Cup-Free Option.

Options 2: Use lift-and-release only for initial treatments, ensuring no hypersensitivity or adverse skin reactions.

For more details about any exceptions, review pages 78–84 in *Chapter 5: Before Beginning Cupping.*

The Cheeks

LOCATION

The cheeks cover a large surface of the face; each cheek extends from above the upper jawline to just under the delicate eye tissue space, and from the side of the nose to in front of the ear.

STARTING POINT

There are typically two starting points here, since the cheek is larger.

The first starting point is at the side of the mouth, where you finish *Step 4: The Mouth Area.*

The second starting point is one cup-width above; it is located at the side of the nose, directly over common sinus points. Many people naturally massage this area next to the nostrils when experiencing sinus congestion.

LINE OF MOVEMENT

There are typically two lines of movement here, since the cheek is larger.

The first line of movement travels along the underside of the cheekbone and ends in front of the ear.

The second line of movement is one cup-width above; it travels directly over the cheekbone and ends in front of the ear, too, one cup-width higher than the first line of movement.

If the face is longer, a third line of movement is possible.

No matter who is receiving treatment and what the shape of their face, the topmost line of movement in the cheek always ends where the upper rim of the cup is just below the delicate eye tissue. That area is treated in *Step 7: The Eyes.*

END POINT

End in front of the ear. You will have at a minimum two end points, one in front of the ear lobe and one just above that, in front of the tragus ear tab.

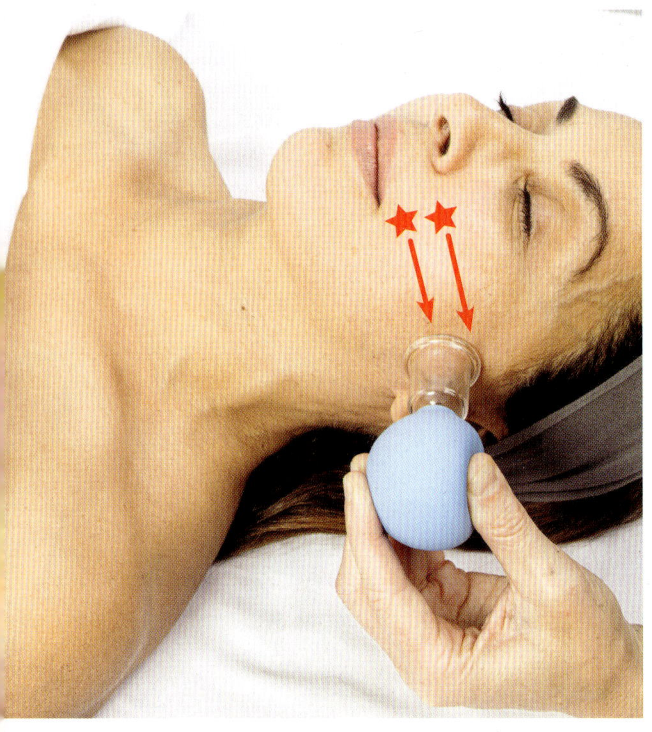

TREATMENT PROCESS

Note: *Be sure you are using a larger cup as you begin the cheek area.*

➤ Attach the cup at the starting point and follow each line of movement using lift-and-release and/or moving cups to the end point(s).

➤ Repeat each line of movement three to five times. In all, you will complete six to ten lines of movement.

➤ Once *Step 5: The Cheeks* is completed, use lift-and-release and/or moving cups to move the cup down the side of the face toward the jump-off location in front of the earlobe, and then follow the Universal Pass **U** one to three times before proceeding to *Step 6: The Forehead*.

If interested, proceed to the Wrinkle-Reduction Option now, before continuing on to *Step 6*. (See page 138.)

The Cheeks

CUP-FREE OPTION

If the cups will not work in this region for whatever reason (facial hair, cosmetic injections, etc.), simply use your fingertips to follow the Cup-Free Option to gently follow the lymph drainage pathways.

TREATMENT PROCESS

Using the same starting points, lines of movement and end points as instructed with cups, use your flattened fingertips to gently create small half-circles across the surface of the skin following the lymph drainage pathways.

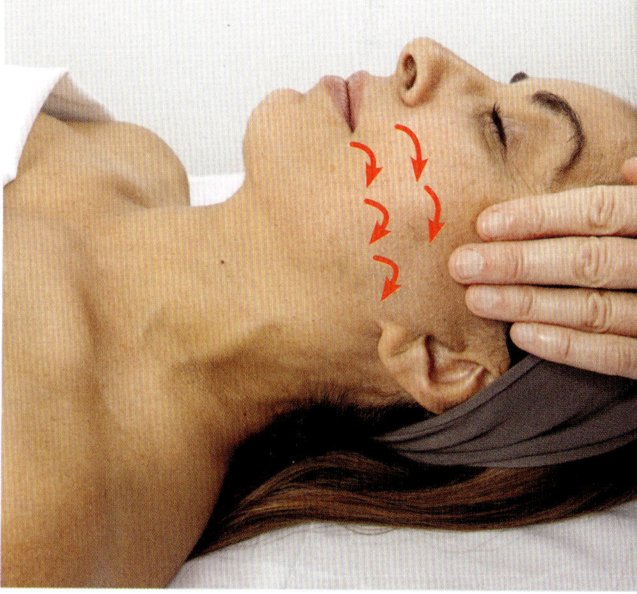

- Use the same hand as the side of the face as you are treating for this Cup-Free Option. When you are working on the left side of the face, use your left hand and progress toward the left ear (as in the photo); when you are working on the right side of the face, use your right hand and progress toward the right ear.
- Begin your fingertip half-circles in the space between the corner of your mouth and the nostril; this is generally where "smile line" wrinkles exist, and where *Step 4: The Upper Lip* just ended.
- Starting at the corner of the mouth, gently use your flattened fingertips to lightly stretch the skin upward and around toward the ear.
- Completely remove your fingertips from the skin after every half-circle is completed, then "step" your fingertips to the next starting place and repeat. Do this until you have covered the entire line of movement across the cheek. The average person's cheek will accommodate three or four placements over each line of movement.
- Repeat each line of movement three to five times.
- Once *Step 5: The Cheeks* is completed, use flattened fingertips to move down the side of the face toward the jump-off location in front of the earlobe, and then repeat the Universal Pass **U** one to three times before proceeding to *Step 6: The Forehead*.

The Cheeks

WRINKLE-REDUCTION OPTION: SMILE LINE WRINKLE REDUCER

CUPPING MARKS POTENTIAL

Remember, any Wrinkle-Reduction Options included in this book has the potential for leaving minor cupping marks, so be sure to visually monitor the tissue as you work.

What we call smile lines are also known as the nasolabial lines. (See page 96 in *Chapter 5: Face Cupping for Cosmetic Rejuvenation*.) This common wrinkle area is formed at the confluence of the many muscles of the face associated with smiling. While you work the cheek area, this is a good location to add some twisting movements for wrinkle reduction.

After finishing the cheek treatment process above, use a smaller cup to revisit this wrinkle area, focusing on the smile lines.

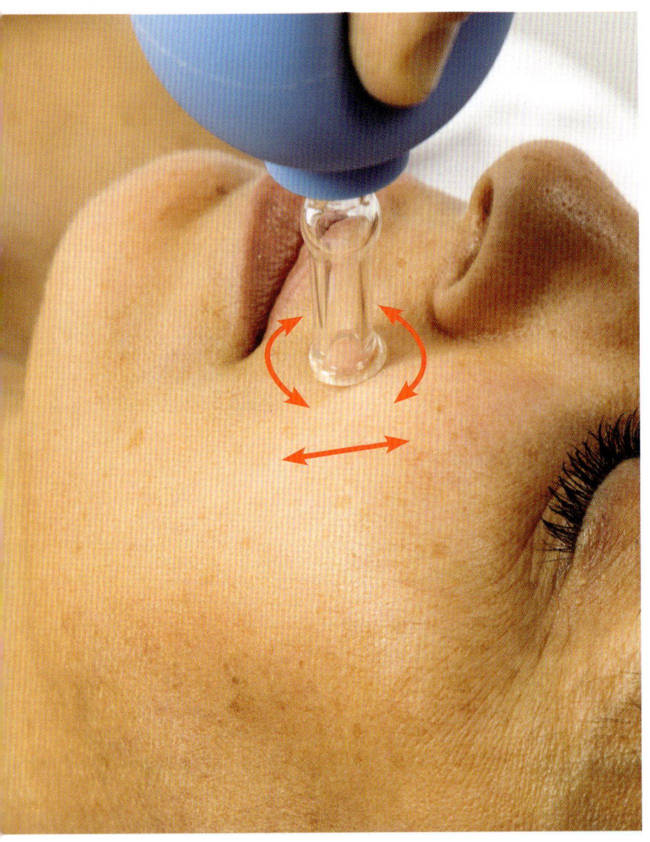

TREATMENT PROCESS

➤ Attach the cup at the top of the wrinkle line, just below the outer rim of the nostril.

➤ Begin twisting the cup back and forth *while* you slide it down the length of the wrinkle, ending at the corner of the mouth.

➤ Repeat this twisting, moving the cup up and down the wrinkle three to five times.

➤ Once finished, repeat a few lines of movement from the center of the upper lip, through the nasolabial wrinkle lines, and across the first line of movement for the cheek area (from the corner of mouth over to the ear). Repeat these additional lines of movement two or three times.

➤ Then repeat the Universal Pass **U** one to three times before continuing to *Step 6: The Forehead*.

Note: *Attach a smaller cup at the top of the wrinkle line to focus on the wrinkle. Once finished, switch to a larger cup and repeat a few lines of movement into the cheek. Try not to pull lip tissue if using a larger cup here.*

The Forehead

The forehead is another large area of the face within which there are several muscles associated with facial expressions, as well as wrinkles and headaches. The largest muscle here is called the frontalis, which travels up the length of the forehead from eyebrow to hairline. Another muscle here, called the procerus, is a very expressive muscle associated with furrowed brows and glabellar lines, or "11s." Also located here are the paranasal sinuses, including the frontal sinuses just above the eyebrows. Important blood and lymph vessels also travel through this region.

WHY CUP THE FOREHEAD?

Cupping across the forehead offers much benefit, both lymphatically and cosmetically. Cupping the forehead relieves sinus congestion, relaxes muscle tension associated with wrinkles or headaches, and gently clears lymph from this often restricted area.

For the greatest benefits, treatment for this section is divided into two parts: *The Centerline*, which follows the sinus drainage area, and *The Entire Forehead* area.

The Centerline. Cupping up this midline should be short and sweet, relaxing and therapeutic. The intention here is to further support lymph drainage from the frontal sinuses located above and around the eyebrows while relaxing muscle tension. And it feels amazing! Whether focusing on acupressure points, the "third eye," the indigo chakra region or simple muscle tension, be sure to take a few moments—maybe encourage your client to take a few deep breaths—while you clear this line of tension.

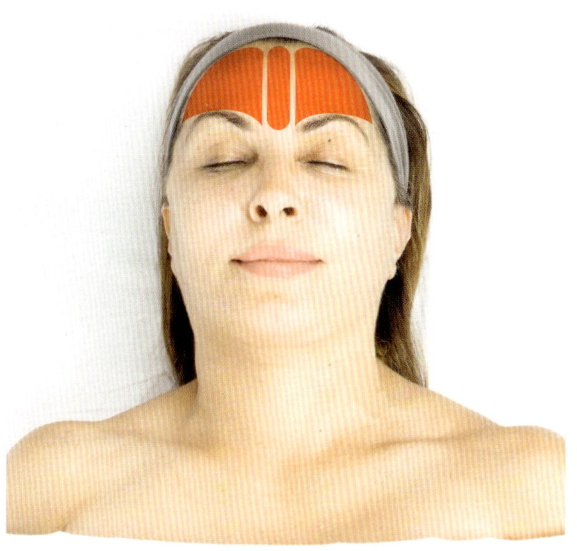

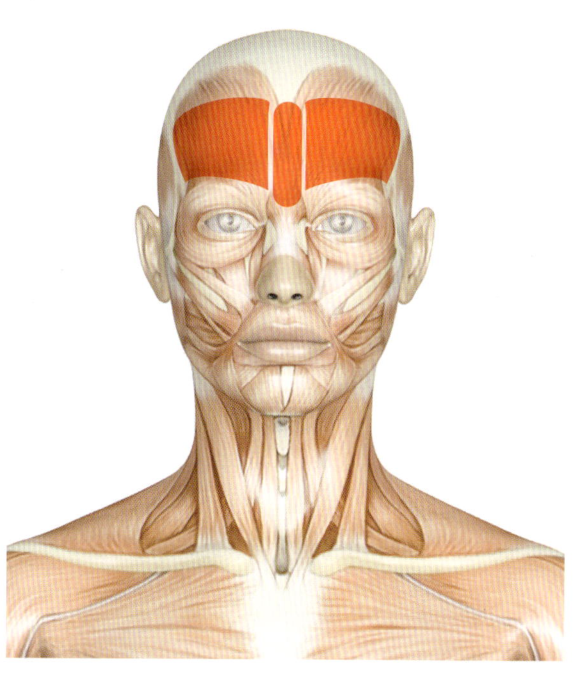

SAFETY POINT

As you work across the forehead, you may encounter veins that are easily visible through the skin; perhaps some may even protrude. Be sure to skip over these veins to the best of your ability. If there are too many veins to make this an easy application, either use only the lift-and-release technique to skip your way through the region, or simply use your fingertips to follow the Cup-Free Option.

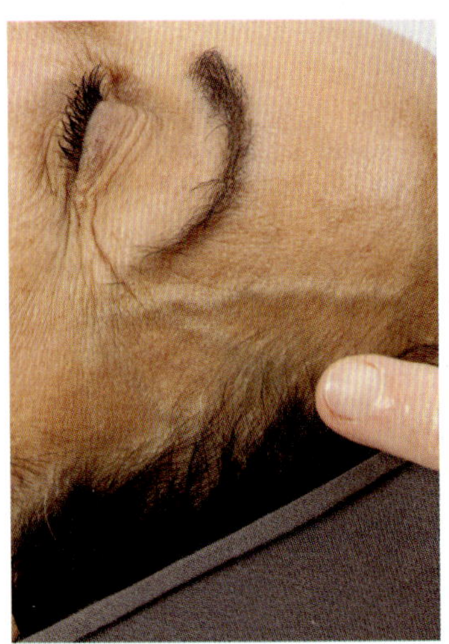

Visible blood vessels
in temporal region

The Entire Forehead. Cupping across the entire forehead addresses the rest of the area at the top of the face, from hairline to eyebrows. Cupping along these horizontal lines follows general blood flow while simultaneously supporting the lymph drainage as it moves across the forehead, toward the temple area, down the side of the face and into the lymph nodes in the neck. Additionally, cupping across the forehead massages the frontalis muscle in a cross-fiber, relaxing manner. Wrinkles that form here will ease as the cupping relaxes muscle tension, and with cumulative treatments, cosmetic benefits are observed.

CUP CHOICE AND USE

Regardless of its size, the forehead is another large area of the face, so you should use a larger cup to treat it. While this is the ideal approach, it may be challenging if there is a lot of tension or there are bony ridges or prominent veins.

First, try to gently use lift-and-release across the forehead to avoid any awkward attempts at moving cups.

If a larger cup still is not easily used, you may consider using a smaller cup, but be aware that smaller cups can easily mark this larger, vascular surface area due to the focused suction.(See page 60 to learn about potential cupping marks on the face.)

If neither cup option works easily, use the Cup-Free Option to treat the forehead.

In my experience, I have seen bodyworkers express frustration when learning to treat the forehead with cups. This can lead to either cupping marks or aggressive placements—strong pressing—into the face, which is not only counterproductive but also yields less-than-pleasant sensations to the recipient.

EASY DOES IT!

Foreheads hold a lot of tension, so consider using the lift-and-release technique across the entire region, including the centerline, if you have difficulty attaching a cup, or if the moving cup encounters speed bumps along any line of movement. If lift-and-release will not work either, follow the Cup-Free Option for initial treatments. These alternate methods of application will not irritate the delicate facial tissues here, which could potentially leave cupping marks.

If this is your experience, consider using these gentle alternatives for the first few treatments, knowing that over time the skin will soften and any subsequent cupping treatments will work toward softening of the region. Remember, some of the best cupping results are cumulative. Often the first cupping application across such tight areas can be challenging. Since great cupping benefits are cumulative, the second or third application can be easier, eventually making for a smoother treatment across the forehead.

WRINKLE-REDUCTION OPTIONS

For the forehead, if desired, you can add in two wrinkle-reducing options: *The Forehead Lift* and *The Glabellar Lines Reducer*. See pages 47 and 148. This is a great location to use the twisting technique (in several directions) as well as the two-cup tension hold. (See page 56 for full descriptions of these techniques.)

After you have completed *Step 6* across the entire forehead, you can apply these wrinkle-reducing, focused techniques.

Note: *When twisting cups, repeat each line of movement one to three times only; be sure to end any cupping if the skin becomes red. (Pink is good circulation; red can be capillary overstimulation and result in cupping marks.)*

> For an additional treatment you might want to offer a bald client, see page 149.

Exceptions

ACNE?

Option 1: Follow the Cup-Free Option.

Option 2: Use lift-and-release as you encounter any acne; moving cups are not recommended. If any blemishes should "pop," cease working over that area for the remainder of the treatment.

RECENT INJECTIONS?

After thirty days post-injection, there are two options:

Option 1: Follow the Cup-Free Option.

Option 2: Use lift-and-release only for initial treatments, ensuring no hypersensitivity or adverse skin reactions.

For more details about any exceptions, review pages 78–84 in *Chapter 5: Before Beginning Cupping.*

The Centerline

LOCATION

This area addresses a straight vertical line in the center of the forehead.

STARTING POINT

Start in between the eyebrows.

LINE OF MOVEMENT

Move from the center of the eyebrows, above the top of the nose, straight up the centerline of the forehead (unless there are prominent veins), ending at the top of the forehead.

END POINT

End at the top of the forehead, where the hairline naturally begins.

VASCULAR CONSIDERATION

If the frontal supratrochlear veins are prominent, simply attach your cup a little off to the side of the centerline and travel alongside the visible veins for similar effects.

TREATMENT PROCESS

➤ Attach the cup at the starting point and follow the line of movement using lift-and-release and/or moving cups to the end point.

➤ Address this line of movement three to five times.

➤ There is no need to do the Universal Pass after this small area is finished. Once this section is completed, continue to the next part of *Step 6: The Entire Forehead*.

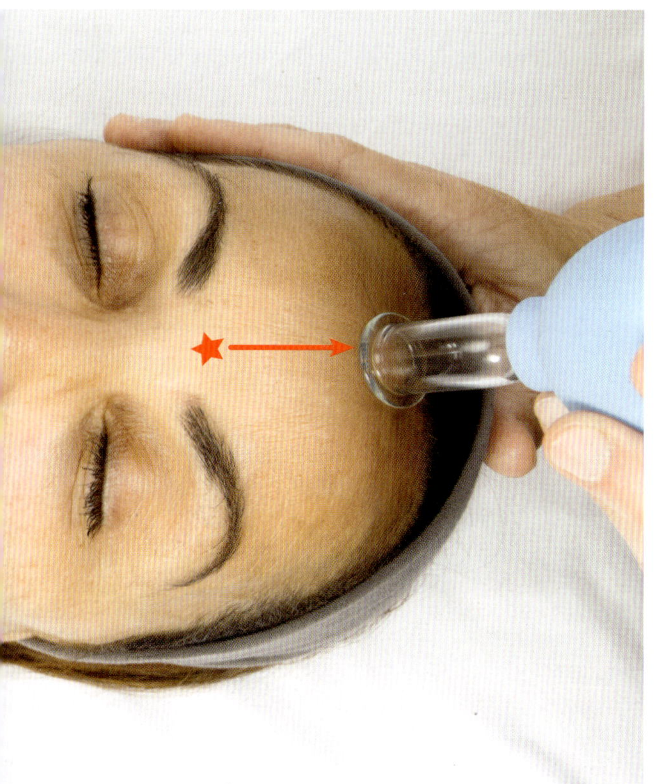

The Centerline

CUP-FREE OPTION

If the cups will not work in this region for whatever reason (tight muscles, recent injections, etc.), simply use your fingertips to follow this Cup-Free Option to gently follow the lymph drainage pathways.

TREATMENT PROCESS

Using the same starting point, line of movement and end points as instructed with cups, use your fingertips to create small half-circles across the surface of the skin.

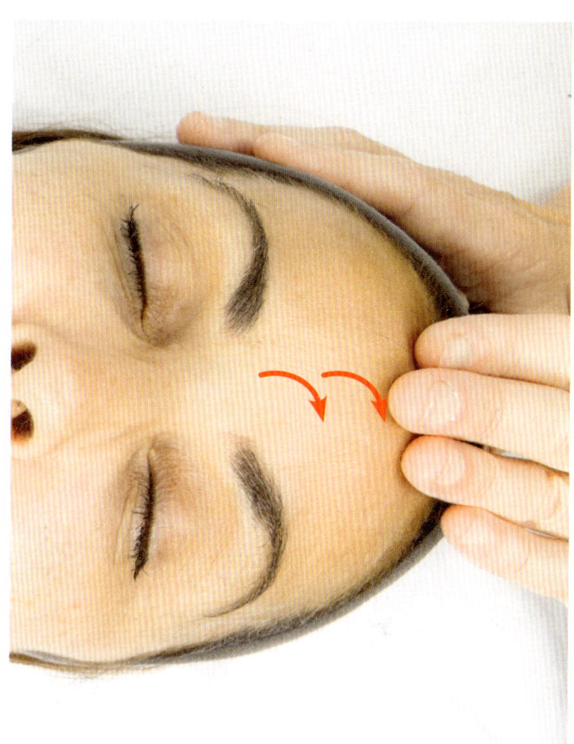

- ➤ Use the same hand as the side of the face you are treating for this Cup-Free Option. When you are working on the left side of the face, use your left hand and progress up toward the hairline (as in the photo); when you are working on the right side of the face, use your right hand and progress up toward the hairline.
- ➤ Begin your fingertip half-circles in the center of the forehead, in between the eyebrows and above the nose.
- ➤ Completely remove your fingertips from the skin after every circle is completed, then "step" your fingertips to the next starting place and repeat. Do this until you have covered the entire line of movement. The average person's centerline will accommodate three or four hand placements.
- ➤ There is no need to do the Universal Pass after this small area is finished. Once this section is completed, continue to the next part of *Step 6, The Entire Forehead*.

SAFETY POINT

Remember: The temple area of the face is considered an endangerment site. If any prominent blood vessels are present, detach the cup completely and skip over them as you proceed.

The Entire Forehead

After the first part of *Step 6, The Centerline*, is complete, you will treat the second part, *The Entire Forehead*. Begin at the top of the forehead where the forehead meets the hairline. Your first line of movement will be at the topmost part of the forehead, progressing one cup-width at a time down the forehead, ending this section above the eyebrows.

Some people have smaller foreheads where you may only be able to fit one or two cup-widths; others have larger foreheads where three or four cup-widths may be accommodated. If the person is bald, begin this step where the hairline would exist.

Remember to use the largest cup possible over this larger surface. If needed, use lift-and-release to facilitate movement across the forehead. Alternatively, if choosing to use a smaller cup, be sure to monitor for redness, since a smaller cup creates more focused suction, possibly more easily creating cupping marks.

LOCATION
This area includes the entire forehead, from the natural hairline down to the eyebrow.

STARTING POINT
Start in the center of the forehead, at the natural hairline.

LINE OF MOVEMENT
Move from the center of the forehead, traveling out to the side (left or right respectively), ending at the temple area.

END POINT
End at the side of the forehead, progressing down toward the temple area and side of the eyebrow.

TREATMENT PROCESS

- ➤ Attach the cup at the starting point(s) and follow the line(s) of movement using lift-and-release and/or moving cups to the end point(s).
- ➤ Repeat each line of movement three to five times.
- ➤ Once *Step 6: The Forehead* is completed, use lift-and-release and/or moving cups to move the cup down the side of the face toward the jump-off location in front of the ear, then repeat the Universal Pass **U** one to three times before proceeding to *Step 7: The Eyes.*

If interested, proceed to the Wrinkle-Reduction Options now, before continuing on to *Step 7: The Eyes.*

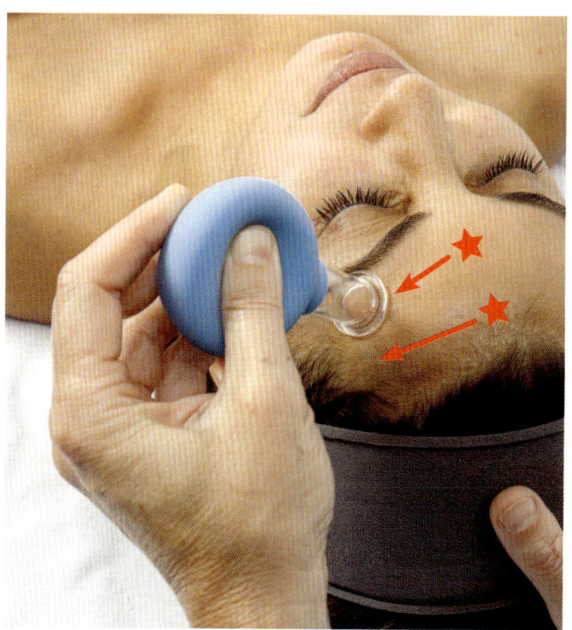

The Entire Forehead

CUP-FREE OPTION

If the cups will not work in this region for whatever reason (tight muscle, cosmetic injections, etc.), simply use your fingertips to follow the Cup-Free Option to gently follow the lymph drainage pathways.

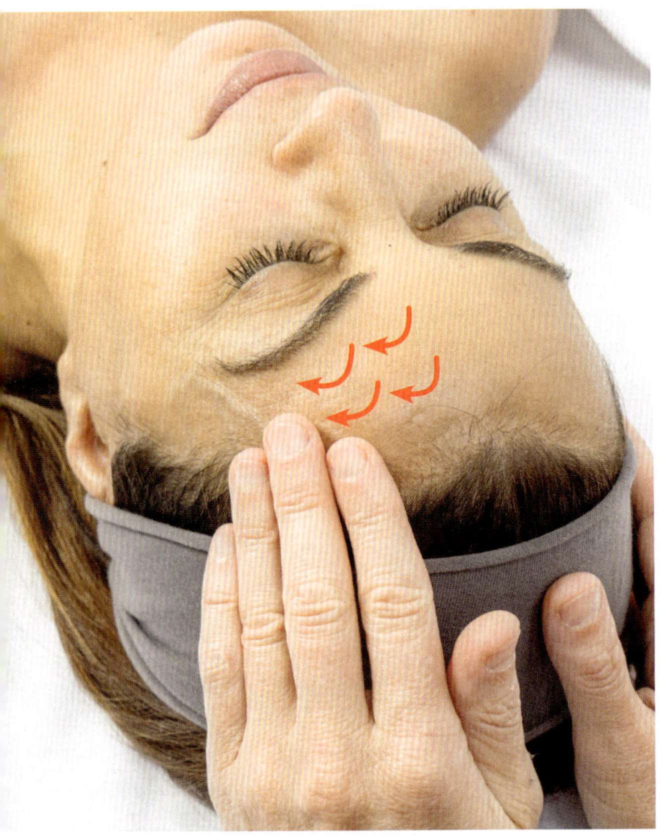

TREATMENT PROCESS

Using the same starting point(s), line(s) of movement and end point(s) as instructed with cups, use your fingertips to create small half-circles across the surface of the skin.

➤ Use the same hand as the side of the face you are treating for this Cup-Free Option. When working on the left side of the face, use your left hand and progress out toward the left temple area; when working on the right side of the face, use your right hand and progress out toward the right temple area.

➤ Begin your fingertip half-circles in the center of the forehead, at the top at the natural hairline.

➤ Starting in the center of the upper forehead, gently use your flattened fingertips to contact the skin's surface and lightly stretch the skin slightly upward and around toward the left side of the forehead.

➤ Completely remove your fingertips from the skin after every half-circle is completed, then "step" your fingertips to the next starting place and repeat. Do this until you have covered the entire line of movement. The average person's forehead will accommodate three or four hand placements over each line of movement.

➤ Once *Step 6: The Forehead* is completed, use flattened fingertips to make half-circles and move down the side of the face toward the jump-off location in front of the ear, then follow the Universal Pass **U** one to three times before proceeding to *Step 7: The Eyes*.

The Forehead

WRINKLE-REDUCTION OPTION: THE FOREHEAD LIFT

The lines that form horizontally across the forehead involve repetitive contractions of the frontalis muscle, often associated with raising the eyebrows. The muscle runs from just above the eyebrows to the top of your forehead where the hairline begins. This option will create length in the frontalis muscle; imagine ironing out these wrinkles as you work across the muscle and possibly upward along its length.

Remember, cupping marks can happen when addressing wrinkles. A little goes a long way.

TWISTING

To address wrinkles across the forehead, use one of the following two twisting techniques: either from side to side along the lines of wrinkles, or from the top of the eyebrows and moving upward toward the hairline to work along the length of the frontalis muscle.

> **Side-to-side twisting cup:** Starting in the center, attach the cup and slowly begin moving it while you twist the cup back and forth. This helps break up adhesions associated with wrinkles, so move slowly and use lighter suction pressure. Repeat each line of movement one to three times only.

> **Upward twisting cup:** Starting above the eyebrow and in the midline, attach the cup and slowly begin moving it upward while you twist the cup back and forth. Travel up toward the hairline, one cup-width at a time, progressing toward the sides of the forehead, ending at the temple area. Repeat each line of movement one to three times only.

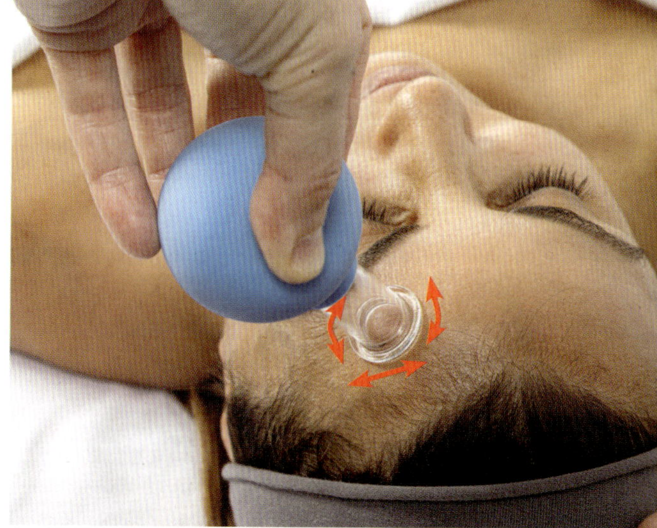

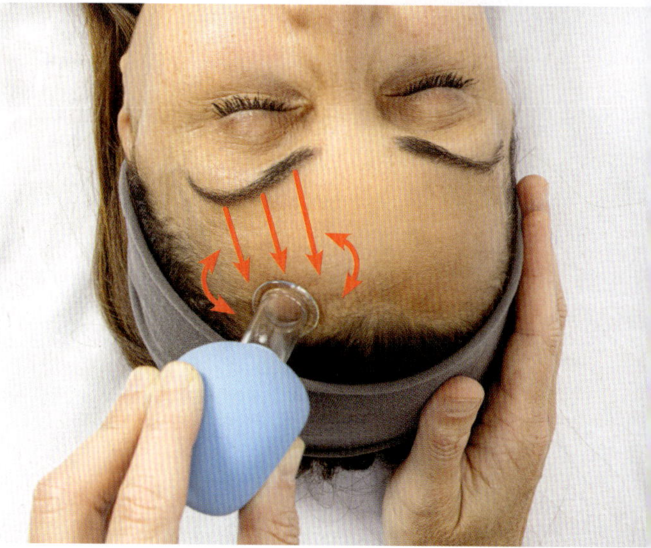

The Forehead

WRINKLE-REDUCTION OPTION: GLABELLAR LINES REDUCER

The lines in between the eyebrows—sometimes called the "11s" wrinkles—involve repetitive contraction of several muscles, including the procerus, corrugator supercilii, depressor supercilii and the medial part of the orbital orbicularis oculi. These wrinkles can be associated with several facial expressions, from laughing and joyous, to worrying or frowning.

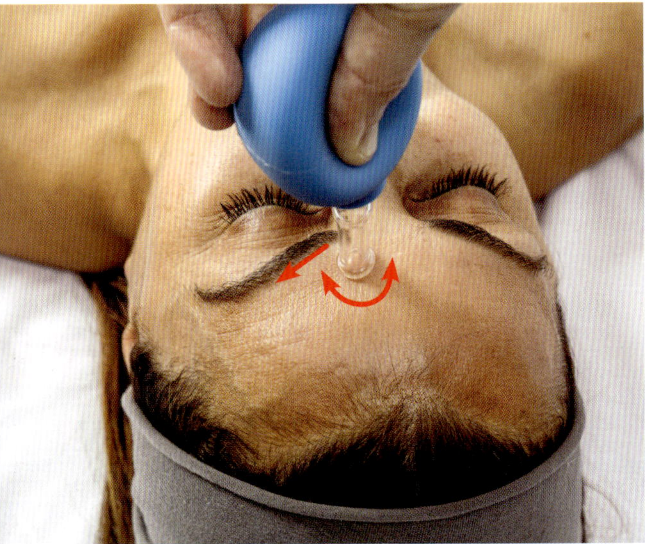

TWISTING

➤ Starting just above the eyebrow and the nose, begin twisting the cup back and forth while you move it along the top side of the eyebrow. Move from the center of the forehead and progress to the sides every time, to maintain the flow of lymph drainage. Repeat each line of movement one to three times only.

TWO-CUP TENSION HOLD

Note: *This add-on is done best after the entire face treatment is completed, both left and right sides of the face. One of the more relaxing techniques, this two-cup technique yields great results.*

➤ Begin by placing two larger cups side-by-side at the center of the forehead, just above the eyebrows. Attach the cups and slowly slide them apart from each other, traveling above the eyebrows, ending at the outer edges of the eyebrows. If using two cups seems complicated, simply use your fingertips to create this tension slide above the eyebrows.

Remember, any Wrinkle-Reduction Options have the potential for minor cupping marks, so be sure to visually monitor the tissue as you work.

Once you have completed the Wrinkle-Reduction Option(s), repeat a few lines of movement from the second part of *Step 6, The Entire Forehead*, working from the center of the forehead, outward toward the temples, down the side of the cheek. Then follow the Universal Pass one to three times before continuing to *Step 7: The Eyes*.

Option: Cupping a Bald Scalp

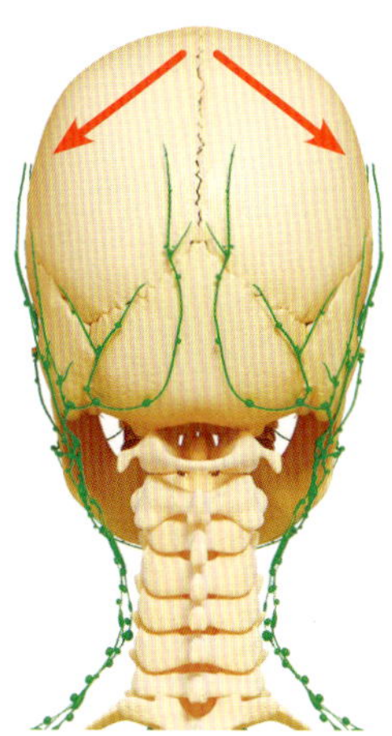

If your client is bald, you may consider adding to their treatment by following the lymphatic drainage pathways over the region, continuing upward and over the top of the skull as you follow along the first part of *Step 6, The Centerline*.

Progressing to the top of the head, move the cup directly along the midline, over the sagittal suture line of the skull, then drain to the left and right side toward the ears and occiput as you progress toward the back. The lymph is collected by lymph nodes around the ears and base of skull, then naturally into the neck along with the rest of the face drainage pathways.

The muscles located in the skull hold a lot of tension, too, so be sure to maintain a lighter suction pressure. Use lift-and-release wherever necessary (which is often many locations over a tight skull) to avoid any possible cupping marks.

The Eyes

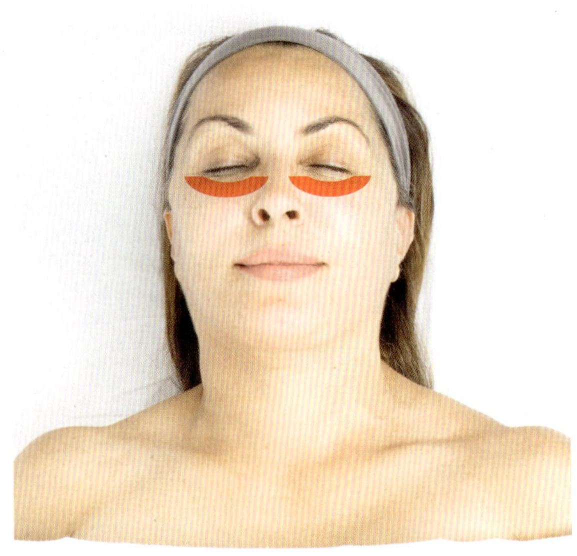

The skin around the eyes is the thinnest, most delicate skin of the entire body. Among the first areas to experience the signs of aging are the eyes, most notably in crow's feet wrinkles at the outer edges, or the bags of loose tissue under and around the eyes.

Because of its fragility, the soft tissue here responds best to gentle manipulation. Any techniques that are more stimulating or invigorating near the eyes will further stretch the tissues, contributing to more wrinkling and loosening. They should be saved for other locations.

Although delicate, the eyes are highly active and involve several muscles, too. There are internal muscles that act on the eyeball itself, and there are facial muscles that affect the area surrounding the eyes.

WHY CUP THE EYES?

While delicate, this area of the face responds very well to gentle cupping. The lightest application can stimulate the underlying capillaries, promoting microcirculation, which will replenish natural collagen and elastin production.

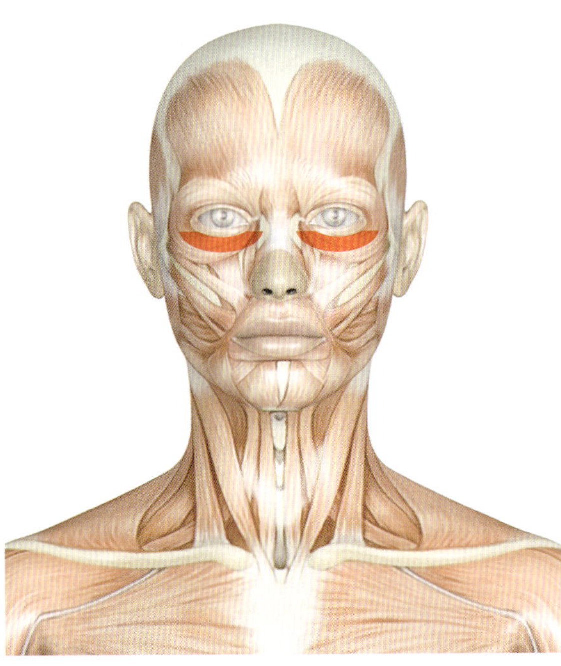

The wrinkles and loose skin around the eyes will respond best to exceptionally light suction pressure, using the lift-and-release technique only. While this is perfectly safe and effective, if you are unsure about approaching this delicate area with your smallest cup, the Cup-Free Option is a wonderful alternative here. This option involves gentle fingertip tapping around the eye area that mimics cupping with lift-and-release. Note that there is also a Wrinkle-Reduction Option for this step.

WRINKLE-REDUCTION OPTION

The crow's feet wrinkles that form at the outer edges of the eyes, technically known as the lateral canthal rhythids, or periorbital lines, are among the first signs of aging to set in. These lines are also known as smile lines, since their formation is generally caused by repetitive contractions of orbicularis oculi muscle, commonly associated with smiling. After you have completed *Step 7*, you can apply this wrinkle-reducing focused technique. See page 154.

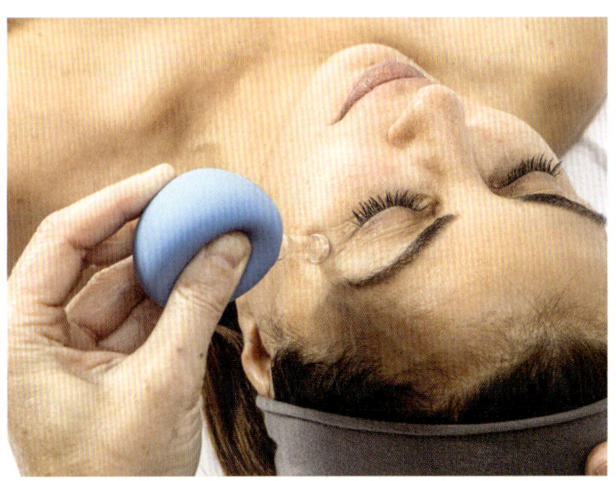

Exceptions

VERY LOOSE SKIN?

With the delicate eye tissue, the only option is to follow the Cup-Free Option.

RECENT INJECTIONS?

After thirty days post-injection, there are two options:

Option 1: Follow the Cup-Free Option.

Option 2: Use very light pressure with the lift-and-release technique, ensuring no hypersensitivity or adverse skin reactions.

Under the Eye

Remember, do not slide the cup in this delicate eye tissue area. No moving cups. Also, do not "extra lift" the cups as you work here. Instead, let the gentle suction of the cup be the only lift of tissue in this delicate region.

LOCATION
This is a very small, delicate region. Be sure to avoid making contact with the lower eyelid near the eyelashes; stay closer to the region at the top of the cheek.

STARTING POINT
Start below the inner corner of the eye; at the side of the nose, just above the cheek area.

LINE OF MOVEMENT
This treatment moves from the side of the nose, along the underside of the eye to the outer corner of the eye.

END POINT
End at the outer edge of the eye, still underneath the eye, at the bottom of the delicate eye tissue area.

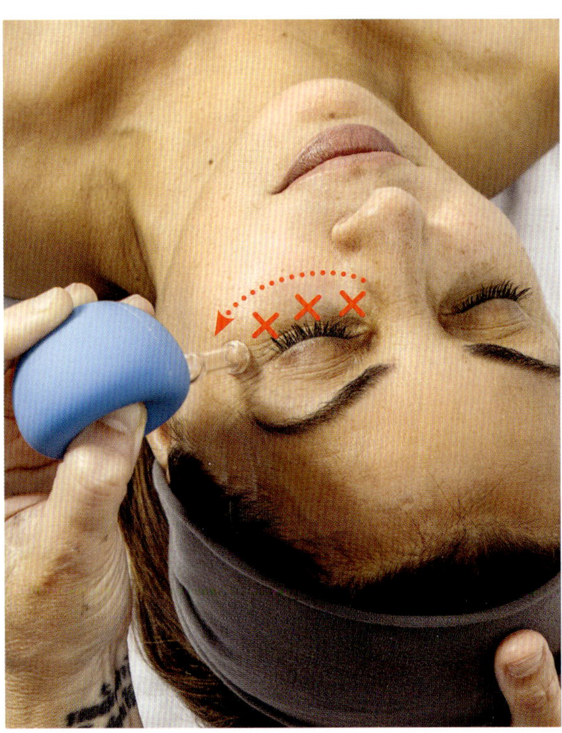

TREATMENT PROCESS
Note: *Be sure to use a very small cup to treat the eye area.*

➤ Attach the cup at the starting point.
➤ Follow this small line of movement using lift-and-release only. Do not use moving cups here.
➤ Repeat this short line of movement three to five times.
➤ There is no need to do the Universal Pass after this small area is finished. Once this section is completed, continue to *Step 8: The Eyebrows.*

If interested, proceed to the Wrinkle-Reduction Option now, before continuing to *Step 8: The Eyebrows.*

Under the Eye

CUP-FREE OPTION

If the cups will not work in this region for whatever reason (facial hair, cosmetic implants, etc.), simply use your fingertips to follow the Cup-Free Option to gently follow the lymph drainage pathways.

Because of the delicacy of the eye area, this Cup-Free Option is highly recommended, very popular and extremely beneficial for everyone.

TREATMENT PROCESS

Using the same starting point, line of movement and end point as instructed with cups, use your fingertips to gently tap along the underside of the eye. We call this method of application the "piano move." This technique is very beneficial for toning the delicate skin here.

➤ Use the same hand as the side of the face you are treating for this Cup-Free Option. When you are working on the left side of your face, use your left hand and progress toward the outer edge of the eye (as in the photo) near the left temple area; when you are treating the right side of the face, use your right hand and progress toward the outer edge of the eye near the right temple area.

➤ Using three or four fingertips, begin your gentle yet quick tapping one fingertip after the other, and progress along the line of movement from the center outward toward the outer edge of the eye.

➤ Repeat this line of movement several times, with as many as ten to twenty rounds of this gentle, fingertip tapping.

➤ There is no need to do the Universal Pass after this small area is finished. Once this section is completed, continue to *Step 8: The Eyebrows.*

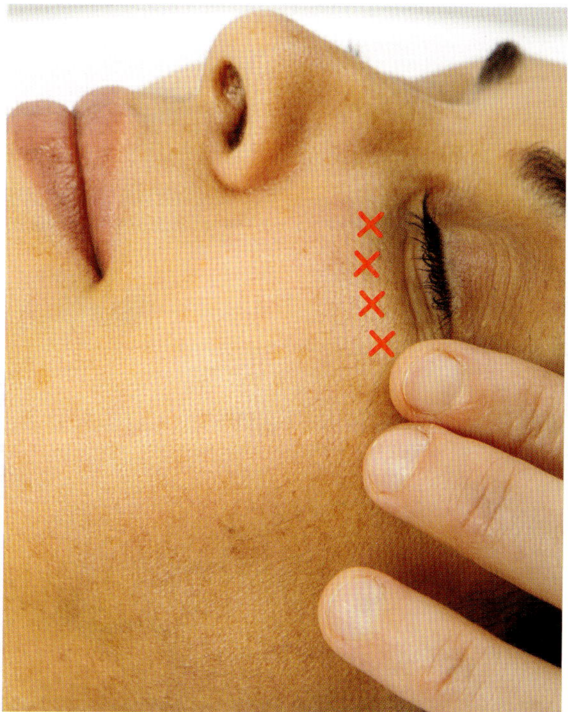

TECHNIQUE FYI

Tapping around the eyes is a form of the percussive massage technique *tapotement*, which offers many levels of benefit to facial tissues. Using fingertips and applied with light pressure, tapping stimulates the diffusion of nutrients at the capillary level, promotes purification of the system by releasing carbon dioxide and other waste materials and helps tone sluggish skin.

The Eyes

WRINKLE-REDUCTION OPTION: CROW'S FEET REDUCER

The best way to address these wrinkle lines is by repetitively applying cups using the lift-and-release technique very lightly across the wrinkles, potentially in two locations.

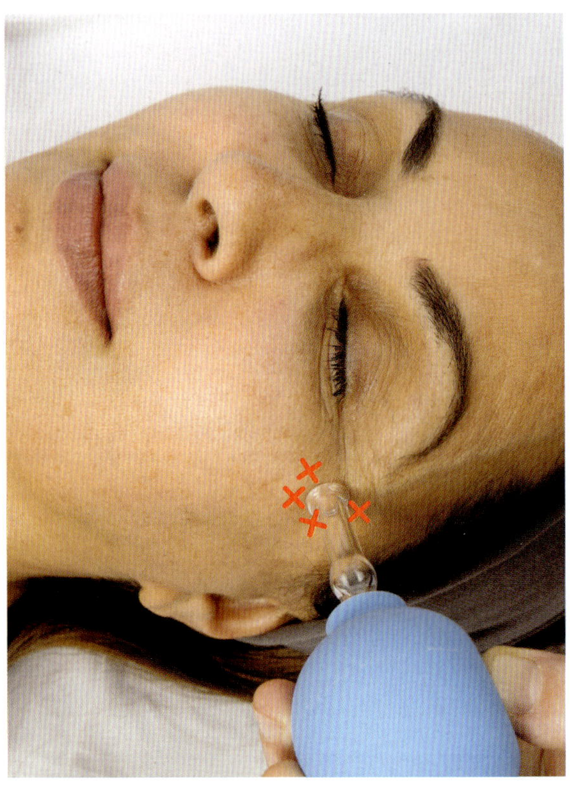

REPETITIVE LIFT-AND-RELEASE

➤ Using very light suction, repetitively apply lift-and-release around the outer edges of the eye, addressing the orbicularis muscle that surrounds the eye.

➤ Using light pressure, apply lift-and-release in the cheek section detailed in *Step 6: The Cheeks*, addressing the zygomatic muscles. (See page 136.) While the orbicularis oculi muscle is the prime moving muscle for these wrinkles, the synergistic actions of the adjacent muscles in the cheek, in particular, the zygomatic muscle, also contribute to wrinkling within this region.

The Eyebrows

Finally, the last section of this treatment involves the eyebrows. This area can hold a lot of tension; tension can originate from the activity of eyes below, the muscles of the forehead above and the paranasal sinuses that are located around them. Fortunately, lots of relief is offered by treating this area.

WHY CUP THE EYEBROWS?

Cupping here wrings out muscle tension in this very expressive area. Additionally, with the decompressive, lifting benefit cups provide, sinus congestion can be greatly relieved. Cupping across the eyebrow also mimics the popular massage technique of "pinching," which is usually done with fingertips. (See the Cup-Free Option.)

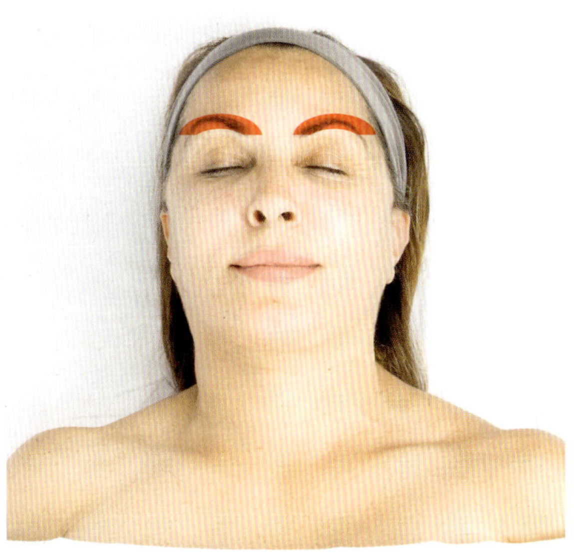

Exceptions

THICK EYEBROW OR BONY RIDGE?

What if the cup does not attach over the eyebrow? If someone has a thicker eyebrow or a prominent supraorbital bony ridge, it may not be possible to encompass the eyebrow with the cup. This is a wonderful opportunity to follow the Cup-Free Option.

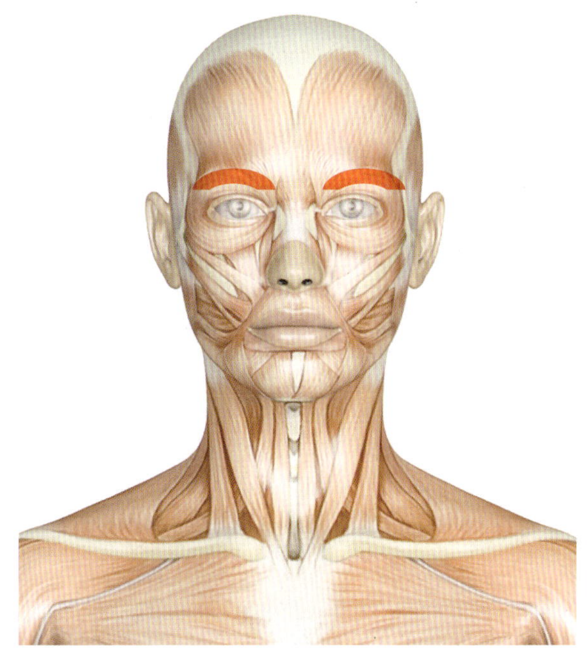

The Eyebrows

Unless there is little to no eyebrow hair, most eyebrows will be lift-and-release only.

Note: *Be sure you are using a cup that fits over the eyebrow; if no cup works, follow the Cup-Free Option.*

LOCATION
This treatment centers directly on top of the eyebrow.

STARTING POINT
Start at the inner edge of the eyebrow, directly above the delicate eye tissue area.

LINE OF MOVEMENT
This treatment moves across the entire eyebrow, from the inner edge toward the temple area.

END POINT
End at the outer edge of the eyebrow, just before the temple area.

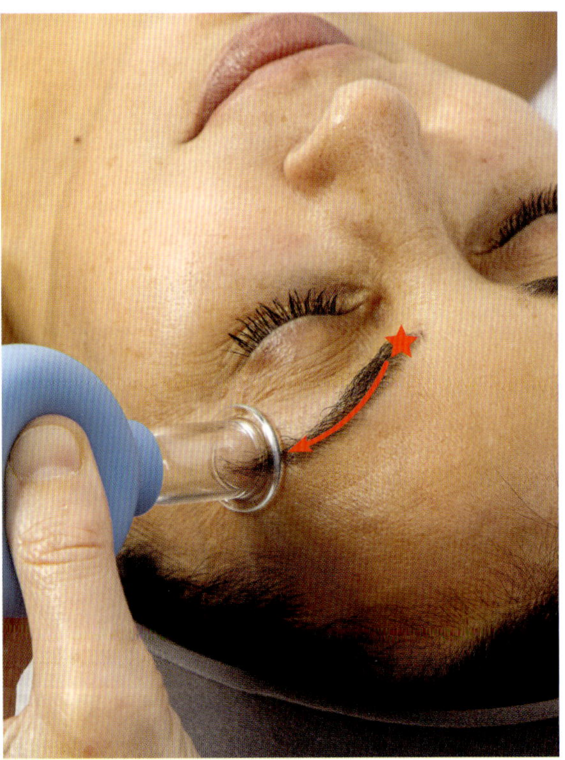

TREATMENT PROCESS
➤ Attach the cup at the starting point.
➤ Using lift-and-release, follow the line of movement across the eyebrow toward the end point.
➤ Repeat this line of movement three to five times.
➤ Once *Step 8: The Eyebrows* is completed, use lift-and-release and/or moving cups to move the cup down the side of the face toward the jump-off location in front of the ear then repeat the Universal Pass **U** one to three times.
➤ Return to *Step 1* and repeat the entire treatment sequence on the right side of the face.

That's it—you have completed the face-cupping treatment.

The Eyebrows

CUP-FREE OPTION

If the cups will not work in this region for whatever reason (facial hair, cosmetic injections, etc.), simply use your fingertips to follow the Cup-Free Option to gently follow the lymph drainage pathways. This option also offers additional sinus congestion relief.

Because of the delicacy of the eye area, and the potential challenge of hairy or bony eyebrows, the Cup-Free Options for treating the eyebrow are highly recommended, very popular and extremely beneficial for everyone.

TREATMENT PROCESS

Using the same starting point, line of movement and end point as instructed with cups, use your fingertips to pinch the eyebrows from the center and progress outward.

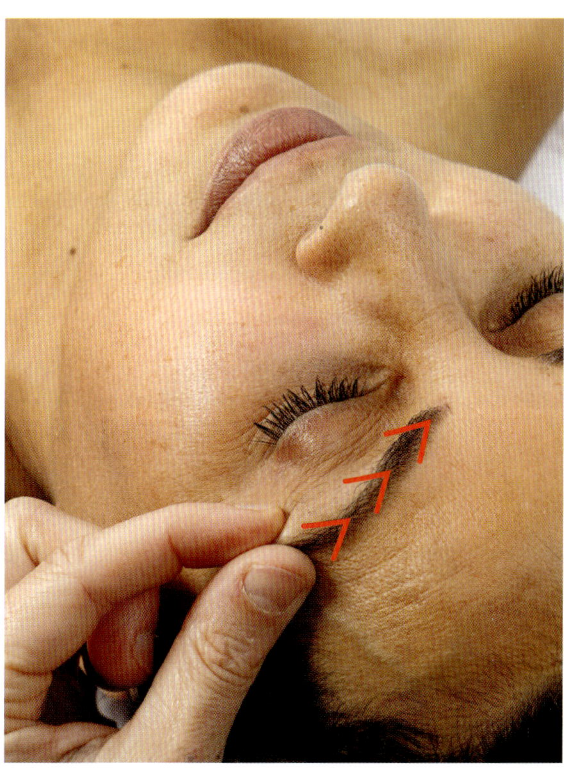

➤ Use the same hand as the side of the face you are treating for this Cup-Free Option. When you are working on the left side of the face, use your left hand and progress out toward the left temple area (as in the photo); when you are working on the right side of the face, use your right hand and progress out toward the right temple area.

➤ Using your thumb and index finger, gently pinch the eyebrows one pinch at a time, progressing out to the side.

➤ Once *Step 8: The Eyebrows* is completed, use flattened fingertips to make half-circles and move down the side of the face toward the jump-off location in front of the ear, then repeat the Universal Pass **U** one to three times.

➤ Return to *Step 1* and repeat the entire treatment sequence on the right side of the face.

That's it—whether you used Cup-Free Options or not, you have completed the face-cupping treatment.

THE FACE-CUPPING MAP

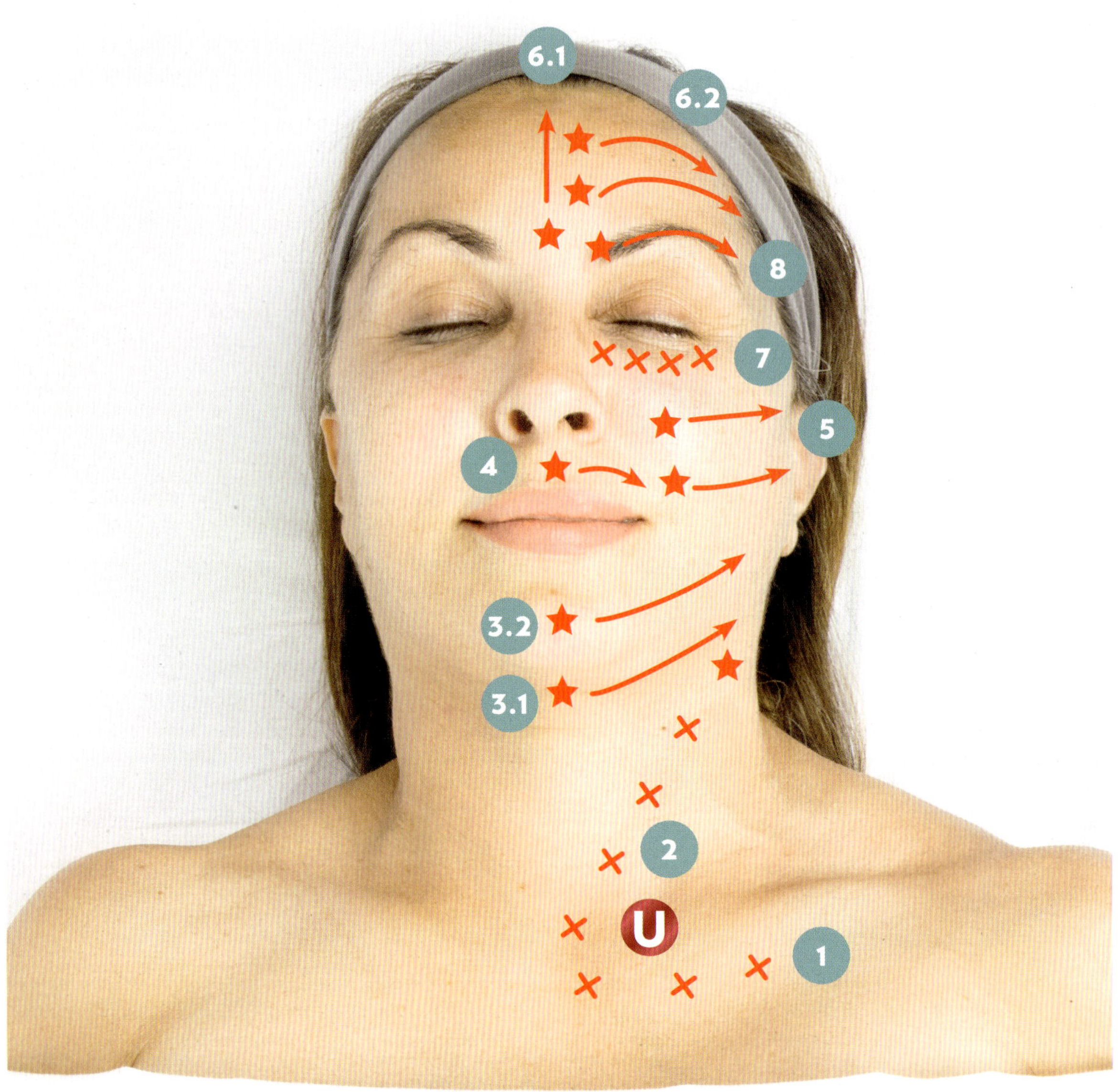

1	**Step 1:** The Upper Chest (page 116)	**6.1**	**Step 6:** The Centerline of the Forehead (page 142)
2	**Step 2:** The Front of the Neck (page 120)		
		6.2	**Step 6:** The Entire Forehead (page 144)
3.1	**Step 3:** Below the Jawline (page 124)	**7**	**Step 7:** The Eyes (page 152)
3.2	**Step 3:** Above the Jawline (page 126)	**8**	**Step 8:** The Eyebrows (page 156)
4	**Step 4:** The Mouth Area (page 129)	**U**	Universal Pass / Step 1 and Step 2 combined (pages 116/120)
5	**Step 5:** The Cheeks (page 135)		

FACE CUPPING FOR SELF-CARE

As much as you may enjoy offering face cupping to clients, I have no doubt that you will soon discover this is a wonderful treatment to do for yourself! You too can reap the benefits described here.

You can easily follow the step-by-step directions and use the one-page *Face-Cupping Map* as a reminder of what comes next.

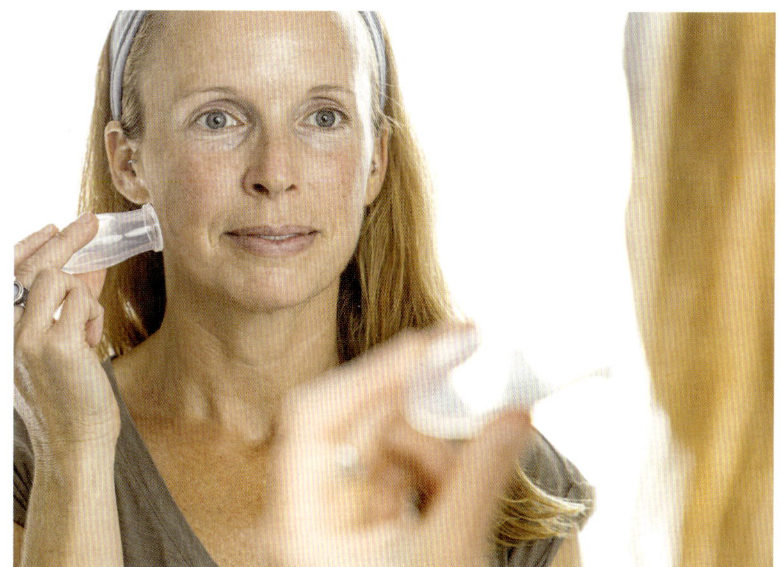

The best way to treat yourself is in front of a mirror. You can see what you are doing and watch how your skin reacts. Moreover, when standing or sitting in front of a mirror to do this, the elevation of your head will further support lymph drainage as it flows down the neck into the upper chest.

Self-care face cupping allows for additional benefits, too.

- First, as a practitioner, you will experience the sensations, and thus be able to sympathize with your clients. Treating yourself will allow you to make comfortable adjustments while you are completing the process. This knowledge— knowing what too much suction feels like, or the feeling of not using enough oil, or meeting a restriction and having to switch techniques during the process—can only make for a better treatment for others thereafter.
- Also, since cumulative effects are easily noticed with face cupping, clients who are curious or hesitant will see how the practitioner looks after treatments. Your fabulous results will encourage them to try it for themselves.

I would not be the cupping practitioner or author I am today without the self-care face-cupping treatments I have done for myself over the years. For more about my personal experience, you can turn to the final chapter of this book, *The Full Potential of Therapeutic Cupping for Skin Health: My Story.*

CHAPTER 8

AFTER A FACE-CUPPING TREATMENT

AFTER-CARE RECOMMENDATIONS

Once you have finished the face treatment, there are a few ways to compliment the face-cupping session so your client gets even more out of each treatment. Some of these recommendations may be more suitable for skincare professionals than other professional bodyworkers, but learning how to complement this face-cupping treatment will enhance both immediate results and future expectations.

Cleanse the face. While oil is great for the skin, ideally the face should be cleansed after the face-cupping treatment is completed. Not only does this remove the oil and any pore gunk that may have been loosened and "vacuumed" from the pores, but it also prepares the skin for whatever great products that are applied afterwards.

If you would like to use another warm—not hot—compress after the treatment to remove oil and dirt, or perhaps a cool—not cold—compress to soothe the circulation-boosted area, be sure the temperature isn't extreme in either direction. The face can be cleaned hours later at home, or immediately after the treatment.

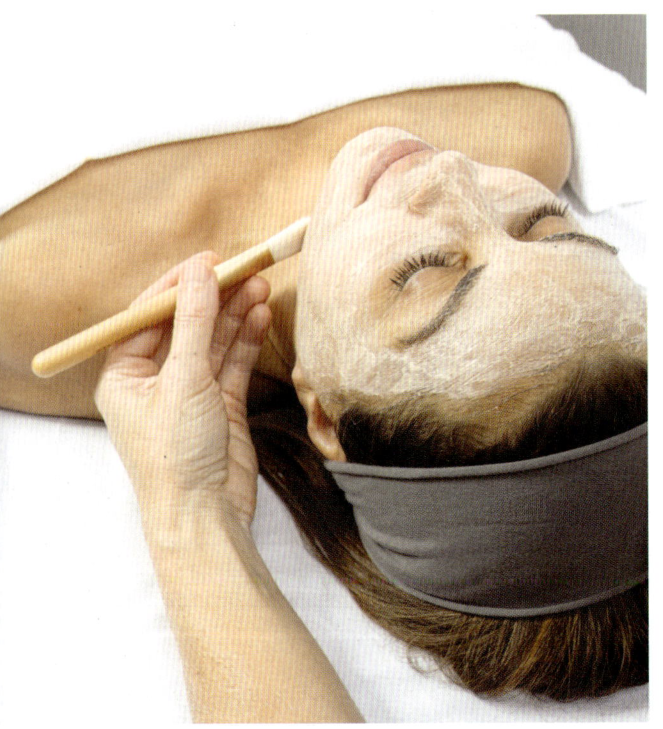

Apply favorite skincare products. Since cupping boosts circulation and gently dilates the pores, as circulation recedes, any product applied afterward will be absorbed more efficiently. Whether applying a favorite serum, quality face oil or a good moisturizer, any product chosen will have a more penetrating effect when applied immediately following the face-cupping treatment.

Option: Apply a face mask! Thanks to the boosted skin activity that follows cupping, what better time to use a cleansing, tightening or toning face mask? Skincare professionals enjoy incorporating face cupping into their routines, as its benefits are easy to observe. After the mask application has ended, apply a favorite skincare product to complete the treatment.

MAKE A TREATMENT PLAN

How often can someone receive a face-cupping treatment? I recommend that treatment is done no more than every 48 hours. While the results are amazing, if this were to be done every day, some adverse reactions could occur.

First, since cups affect fluid levels in the tissues, cupping too much could create swelling. And if this swelling persists, over time it could cause circulation issues. Furthermore, if it occurs repeatedly, the skin could become distorted, causing it to sag.

Also, if the face is cupped daily, it will most likely result in cupping marks. Leave 48 hours between treatments to allow the circulation of fluids and the muscles and fascia to fully process the treatment.

Still interested in daily treatments? For an alternative, full-face treatment, consider following the eight steps but using the Cup-Free Options only. Since manual lymph drainage is safe to experience every day, this is a wonderful option for daily usage.

Scheduling Recommendation: Pick one or two days maximum per week to schedule a treatment. In clinical practice, scheduling a face-cupping treatment is great as an add-on service done at the end of a session. For self-care, try to set time aside for yourself, too; I personally aim for "Wellness Wednesdays" as my weekly commitment to myself.

Cumulative Planning Option: For best results, consider scheduling a treatment series. Plan once or twice per week (maximum) for three to four weeks to allow for the greatest, cumulative results to take place. Be sure to take photos before and after the series; you and your client will see (and feel) some wonderful changes, motivating you to keep doing cupping! In my clinical practice, this is a regular add-on service for existing clients, as it is a lovely way to end any therapeutic bodywork session. I also frequently offer treatment series for those planning for special events (weddings, reunions). However you incorporate it, facial cupping is an extraordinary treatment to be enjoyed by all.

FAQ

HOW LONG DO THE RESULTS OF FACE CUPPING LAST?

This is a question you may hear regularly, especially from first-time recipients.

Every person will have different results, and cupping results are most responsive when you follow all recommendations for application, timing and frequency. Cupping results are cumulative and lasting. Yes, the clock of time keeps ticking forward, but with regular treatments, face cupping is one of the most effective, natural treatments to ensure a long, beautiful life of the face.

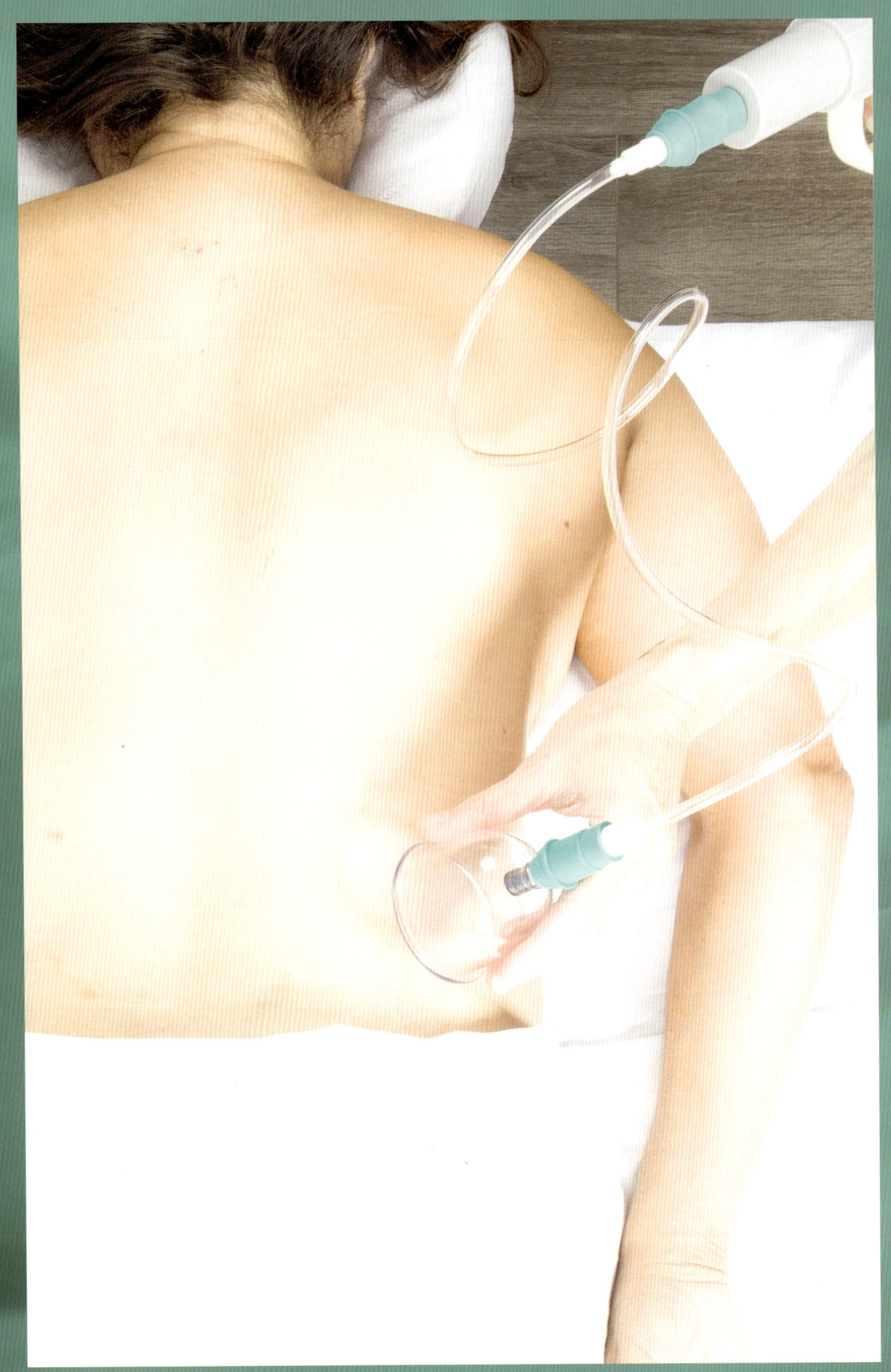

PART III

BODY CUPPING

CHAPTER 9

BODY CUPPING FOR CELLULITE REDUCTION AND CONTOURING

ANATOMY OF CELLULITE

SAFETY POINT

As a general guideline, if someone can receive therapeutic massage and bodywork, they can receive therapeutic cupping. Similarly, anything that contraindicates having massage and bodywork also contraindicates therapeutic cupping applications.

Deciding whether any person can receive the cupping treatments as described in this book will depend on the professional assessment of the bodyworker and their methods of client evaluation. The treatment described in this section is for generally healthy people.

Cellulite is generally defined as dimples created by fat deposits stuck under the skin's surface. While it may be predominantly an issue of unattractiveness, cellulite involves soft tissue dysfunction, circulation challenges and, in some cases, it may include pain. In other words, when cellulite exists, there are many issues present that can affect—and distort—the entire body system.

The puckering on the surface is a result of *adhesions* that form when the more superficial fascia gets "sticky," restricting mobility between skin, fascia and muscle.

Yes, *fascia* is the connective tissue that is intertwined throughout the entire body. In different locations of the body, however, fascia has different compositions. There is structural or subcutaneous fascia (the most superficial fascia, just below the skin's surface), interstructural fascia (woven throughout the entire body), visceral fascia (envelops the visceral organs) and spinal fascia (involved in the spinal column and its anatomy).

CELLULITE ADHESIONS CAN CAUSE RESTRICTIONS AND SYSTEMIC DYSFUNCTIONS

Wherever the adhesions associated with cellulite form, these areas of "stuck" soft tissue increase restriction of body movements and add to systemic dysfunctions.

- **These adhesions can disrupt systemic circulation of blood and lymph.** Blood and lymph travels through fascia and if the fascia becomes restricted, circulation is hindered. If circulation is challenged, soft tissues get dehydrated, which can contribute to more adhesions forming, and in that way the cycle will continue. With restrictions in circulation, the skin can't get all the blood, oxygen and nutrients it delivered by circulatory vessels, nor can the system remove lymph. This causes the health and appearance of skin to diminish.
- **Collagen production is also lessened, and elastin does not receive the oxygen it needs to thrive.** Collagen and elastin help skin keep its original shape, and without proper circulation, they cannot do their cosmetic jobs.

- **Restrictions in fascia can also affect the nerves.** Miles of nerves weave throughout the body, running alongside every blood and lymph vessel. When fascial restrictions cause nerve distortion, this can create various levels of dysfunction. With nerve dysfunction comes interrupted muscle functions (since nerves tell muscles how to operate). If muscles can't contract properly, blood and lymph cannot flow efficiently, which inevitably further inhibits muscle health; on a cosmetic level this can cause the skin to sag.

- **If nerves are stuck in an irregular pattern, the nerve endings at the skin's surface can get stuck in a state of irritation.** That is why many people with cellulite experience pain when touched or manipulated over these perpetually sensitive locations. Some severe cases of cellulite involve low-grade, constant pain, often comparable to fibromyalgia (a systemic condition involving undefined pain sensitivities).

- **Serious fascial adhesions can trigger the central nervous system to protect these comprised areas, thinking they are injuries.** This will cause the nervous system to tighten the fascia even more as it reacts to stabilize and protect this area of soft tissue dysfunction. This vicious cycle of restriction, poor circulation and overall systemic dysfunction will continue unless acted upon therapeutically for correction.

- **When there is cellulite, the adipose (fat) tissue that exists in these surface layers of skin gets sectioned off and clumped together.** As with every other soft tissue structure, adipose tissue thrives when hydrated and supple, freely moving within its anatomical spaces, providing cushioning and nutrient storage. When adipose tissue gets stuck, the skin's surface will bulge and become distorted, adding to the visible dimples and dents.

When all this soft tissue and internal dysfunction is present, the skin can look droopy, saggy, wrinkly and dimply. Upon palpation, the skin can feel cool from challenged circulation or denser where soft tissue pliability is restricted. The internal struggles will show on the surface as cellulite and other cosmetic challenges.

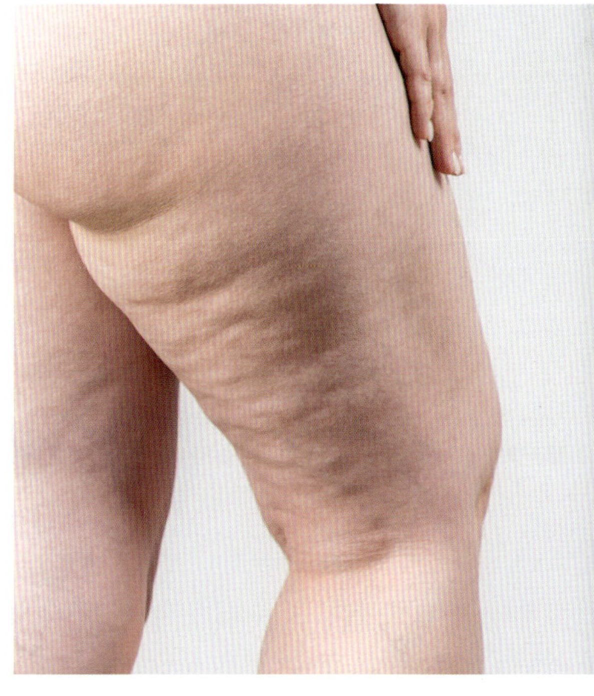

SYMPTOMS AND RISK FACTORS OF CELLULITE

NERVE ENDINGS AND CELLULITE

When cupping for cellulite reduction, you should acknowledge each person's individual response to pressure and sensitivity. If cellulite is present, there can be pain and discomfort if the nerve endings in the surface anatomy are irritated. Furthermore, some people are easily overstimulated with some of the more vigorous, focused applications. Remember, a little cupping goes a long way. Be sure to not cause pain during this treatment process.

These same irritated nerve endings will quickly respond to too much suction pressure, so you should avoid starting with stronger suction. Instead, just as with massage therapy, work slowly into any stronger pressure.

Symptoms of cellulite include both visual and internal components. While cellulite commonly affects the thighs, buttocks, midsection and upper arms, it can affect every body differently. Cellulite can occur for many reasons, too, such as a sedentary lifestyle that contributes to sluggish circulation and muscle tone, a poor diet that lacks nutrition and hydration, or even an unresolved, deep-seated injury. No matter the origin or causes, cellulite is a condition of continuous systemic stagnation and dysfunction.

Common risk factors that contribute to the development of cellulite include:

- **Gender differences.** Cellulite is more common in women, affecting 80 to 90 percent of all adult women. Men have a different collagen structure based on their genetic makeup.
- **Genetic predisposition and body types.** Tendency toward cellulite can be predetermined by one's genetics.
- **Hormonal factors and age.** Cellulite onset occurs after puberty, and its likelihood increases as the body ages, elasticity declines and collagen production diminishes.
- **Dietary and lifestyle factors.** From the foods eaten to the exercises done or not, lifestyle choices play a key role in contributing factors of cellulite.
- **Hydration versus dehydration.** Optimal hydration is beneficial for the overall health of skin, circulation (of blood and lymph) and the suppleness of soft tissues. The interstitial fluid in the extracellular matrix requires hydration to maintain optimal cellular function delivering nutrients, removing waste materials, and so on. On the other hand, if dehydration sets in, tissues get stuck and cellulite sets in. Dehydration can impair fluid movement throughout the body, contributing to the symptoms of cellulite. Dehydration affects interstitial fluids as well, which alters the properties of the fascia, muscle and skin.

BENEFITS OF BODY CUPPING

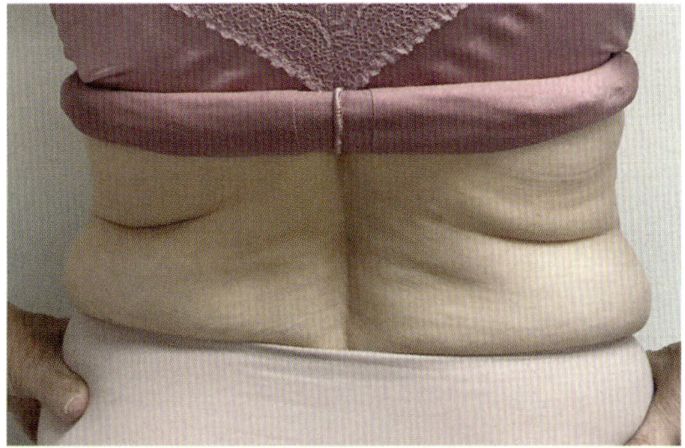

BEFORE

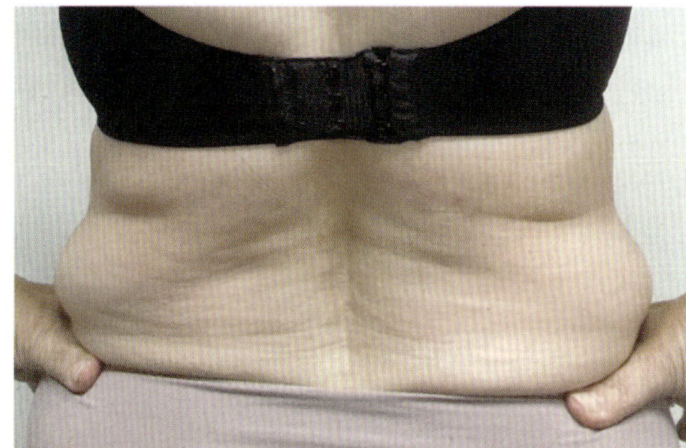

AFTER TWO TREATMENTS

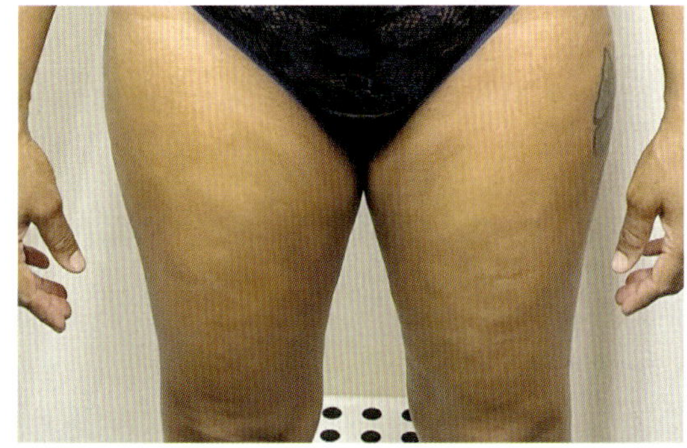

BEFORE

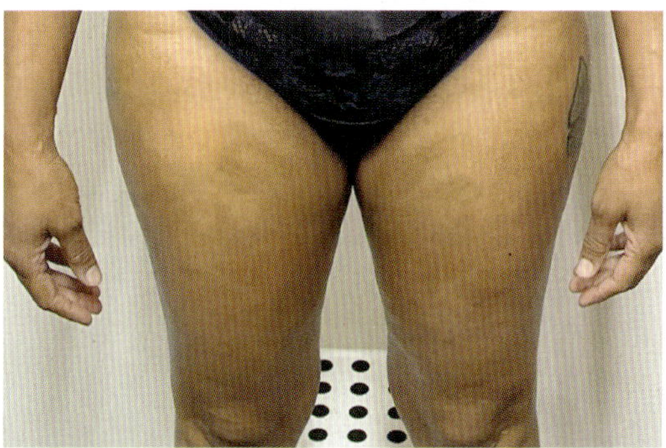

AFTER ONE TREATMENT

Changes in the appearance of cellulite before any body cupping and after treatment.
The client in the top photos has worn compression garments for more than thirty-five years.
After treatments, client felt much-needed softening and contouring in midsection.
The client in the bottom photos suffers from chronic muscular pain in her legs.
After treatment, she noticed immediate relief in addition to cellulite reduction.

We can see the benefits of cupping almost immediately through thermographic images, and we can also see how these benefits continue after the cupping is done.

As explained on page 100, thermographic images show areas of circulatory imbalances. On the following pages, alongside these images, we see photos of the gluteal region and backs of the thighs before, during and after cupping for body contouring has been applied.

In the first images, below, we see the body before starting cupping. Notice the blue indication of cool temperatures, as the gluteal region is the most challenged area of the body when it comes to circulation.

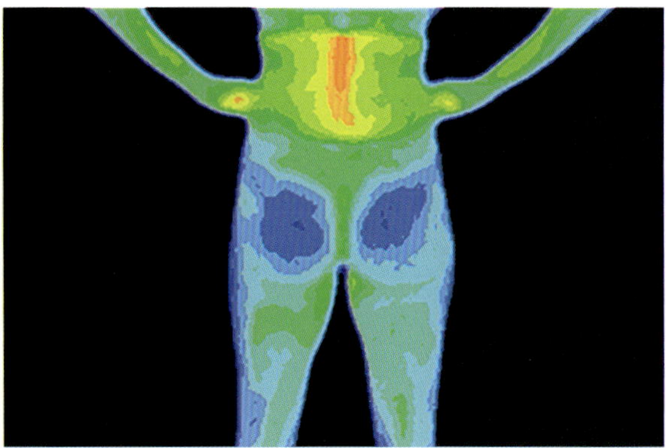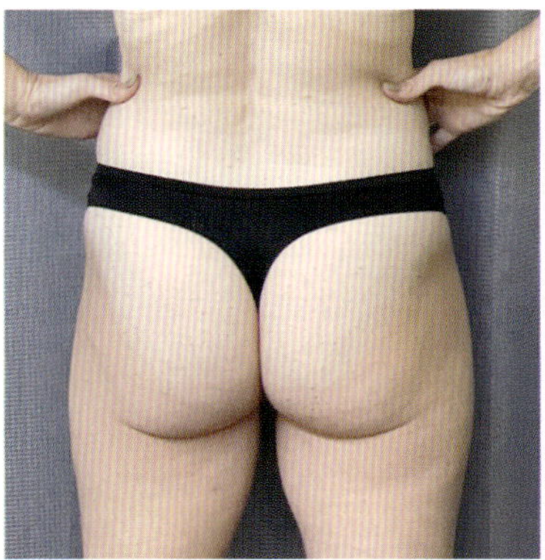

In the second images, we see the left gluteal region has been cupped (the skin is pink, and the client reported some sensitivity as cupping continued), and the accompanying thermographic image shows the boost in circulation.

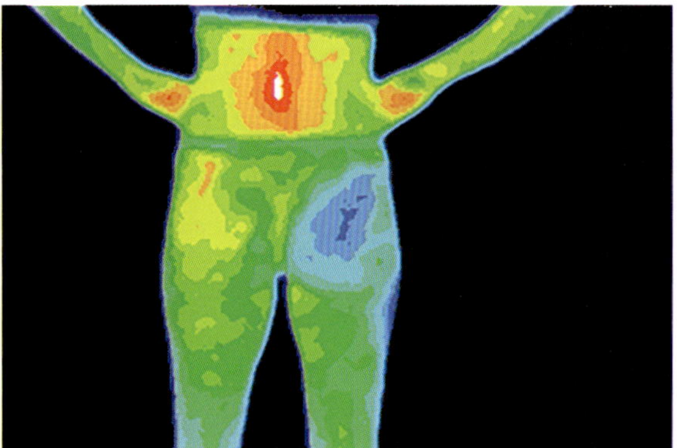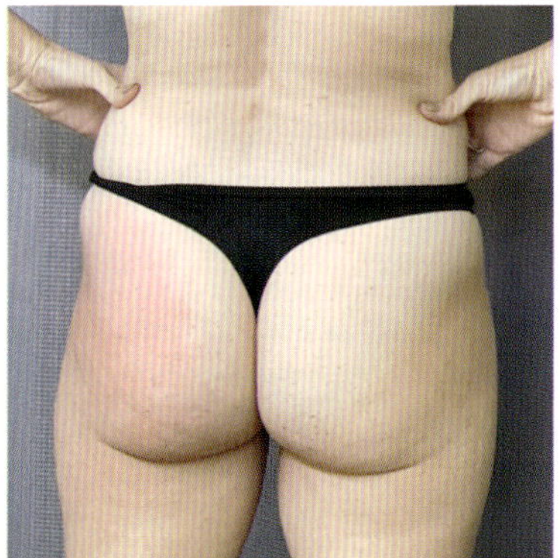

In the third images, we see the right gluteal region similarly completed. The accompanying thermographic shows not only a similar boost in circulation; notice also the continued increase in circulation on the left side. As discussed, cupping enhances fluid-exchange processes. So, when an area is "done" being cupped, the body is still increasing circulation naturally! No need to overwork the client to get such effective results.

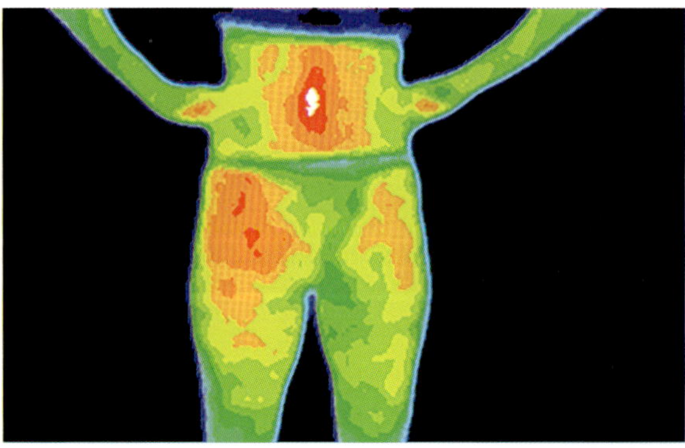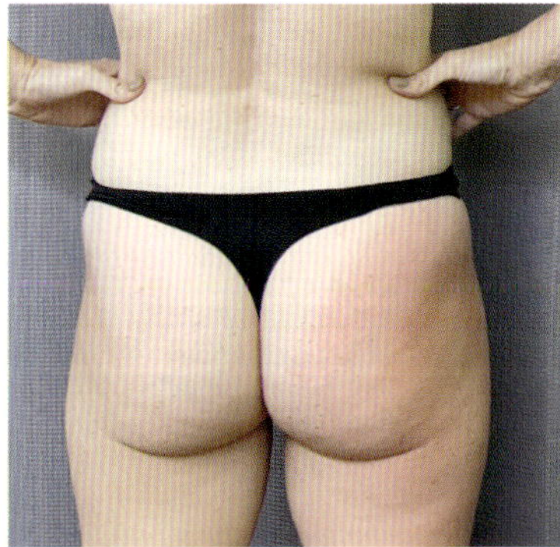

In the fourth images, below, we see both sides completed and a dramatic increase in overall circulation.

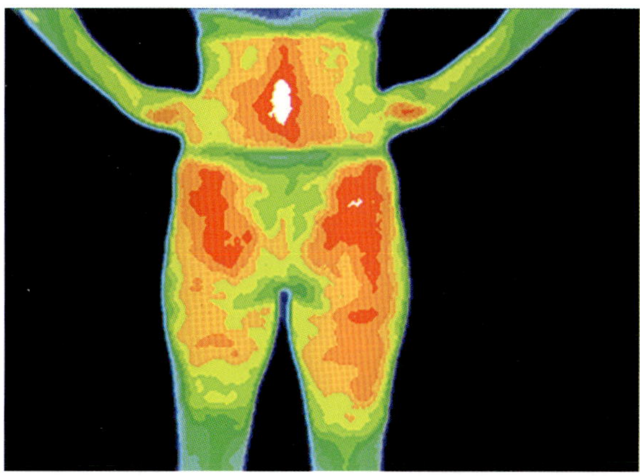 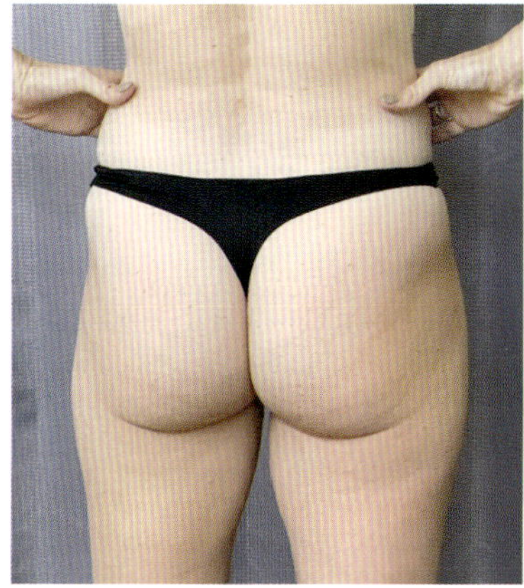

In these final images, we see both sides after given a short period of time to rest. Circulation is evenly stimulated across the region. The client's gluteal region and backs of the thighs felt softer and smoother to the touch as well.

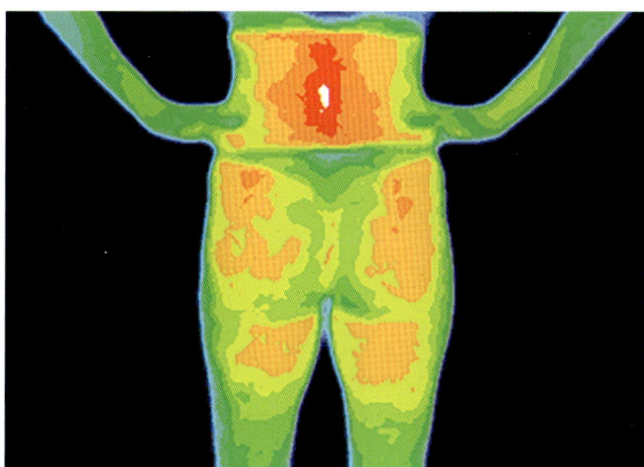 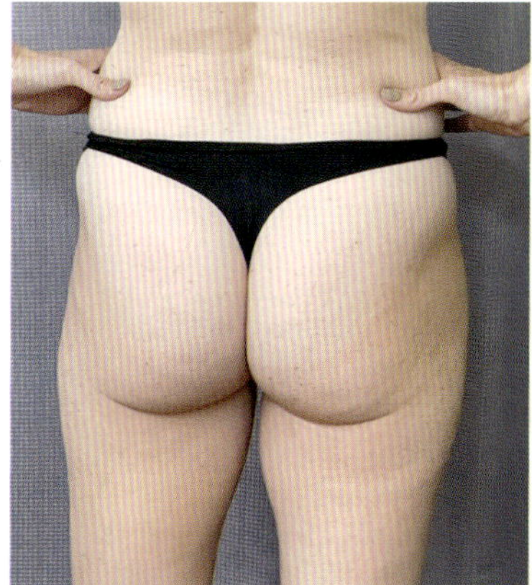

"The glute cupping session yielded outstanding results! It visibly enhanced the firmness and smoothness. I was thrilled with the effect it had on my skin and overall appearance. The treatment also helped alleviate tension and soreness, leaving them feeling much more relaxed. I was pleasantly surprised by how effective it was in targeting this area."

—A satisfied client

LYMPH WATERSHEDS AND PATHWAYS

The lymphatic system follows a specific, intricate route of collection, drainage, filtration and recirculation. For more information, see page 30 in *Chapter 1: The Science of How Cupping Affects the Body.*

- The median watershed divides the torso in half lengthwise (left and right sides); the transverse watershed divides the torso in half through the midsection (top and bottom). The very top of the shoulders and head drain into the supraclavicular region.
- The face and head drain into the cervical lymph nodes, then into supraclavicular nodes, finishing at the thoracic ducts (the left thoracic duct and right lymphatic duct).
- The lower arms drain into the antecubital lymph nodes in the elbow, and the entire arm drains into the axillary lymph nodes.
- The lower leg drains into the popliteal lymph nodes, and the entire leg drains into the inguinal lymph nodes.
- The lower regions of the torso (lower midsection, gluteal region and hips) also drain into the inguinal lymph nodes, while the upper regions of the torso (shoulders, chest, upper midsection) also drain into the axillary lymph nodes.
- The cisterna chyli is a specialized sac of lymph tissue that connects the lower body's drainage to the left thoracic duct.
- The left thoracic duct collects from the lower body, left upper arm and torso and left side of head, while the right lymphatic duct collects from the right upper arm and torso and right side of the head.

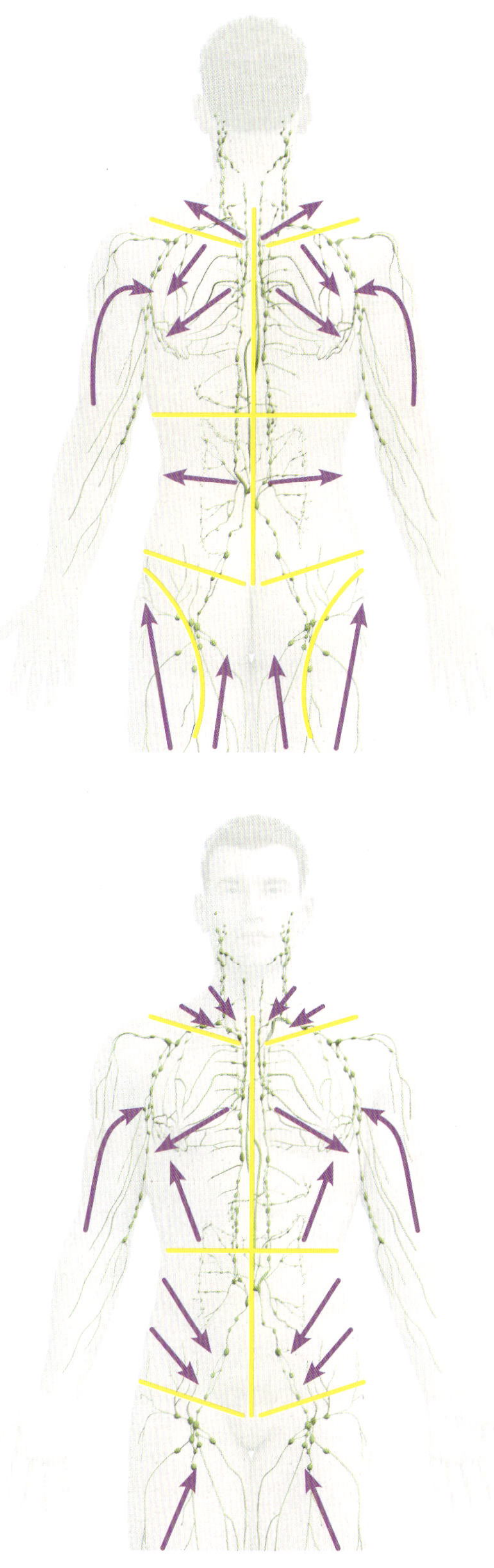

SUPERFICIAL LYMPHATIC SYSTEM

CHAPTER 10

BODY CUPPING STEP-BY-STEP TREATMENT

OVERVIEW OF TREATMENT PROCESS

A TOTAL BODY EXPERIENCE

This body-cupping treatment is intended to address the entire body as one unit and in the specific order in which it is laid out in this book.

The treatment generally follows the lymph drainage pathways of the body, so it follows a systematic, logical method of application. When done correctly, this treatment simultaneously supports lymph drainage while boosting blood circulation. It also reduces muscular tension and alleviates the adhesions between skin, fascia and muscles. This treatment has multi-faceted benefits every time you do it!

WHERE TO BEGIN

When working on both sides of the body, we often work first on one side and then the other. And when the intention is to follow lymph drainage pathways, we follow a very systemic approach, beginning with the core of the body; this is a necessary component of all lymph drainage treatments. In this book, we begin with the left side of the body because the more powerful left thoracic duct is located on that side.

Starting on the left is not required, but that is how it is described here. Whichever side you begin with, what is most important is to be methodical and thorough with this treatment.

Each step of this cupping treatment is designed to address the body as one complete fluid-moving circuit in a logical, holistic manner for greatest efficacy.

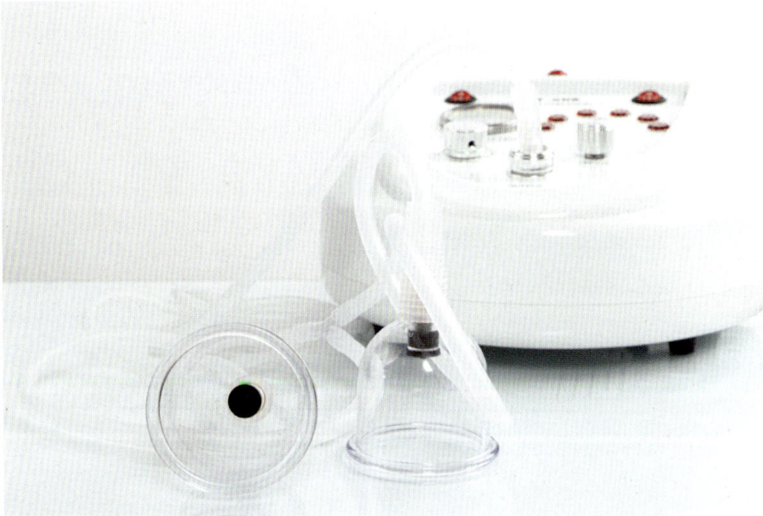

Working both sides of the body simultaneously may be ideal in some instances, but it requires ambidexterity and, usually, a cupping machine with bifurcated hoses and multiple cups. Working one side of the body at a time is just as effective and most comfortable for beginners or self-care.

In this book, the order in which you do the body-cupping treatment is different from the order of the face-cupping treatment. When cupping the face, you first do every step on the left side of the face and then, when the left side is completed, you do every step on the right side. When cupping the body, however, treat each section of the body as it is described for each step, and then move on to the next step when the entire section has been completed. Each step is different from the next, with detailed instructions on how to best address each part of the body.

For example, in *Step 1: The Middle and Lower Back*, you will address this entire region before continuing up to *Step 2: The Back of the Upper Body*.

Whether you address the left side first or the right side first is not as important as it is to complete the entire section before moving on. For the sake of demonstration, all instructions will be described to address the left side of the body first, then the right, one step at a time.

Another example is in *Step 2: The Back of the Upper Body*, where you will stimulate the left axillary lymph nodes, then address the left posterior shoulder, then the left upper arm, and then repeat the entire *Step 2* sequence on the right side of the upper body. And then, before continuing to *Step 3*, you will do the *Finishing the Back of the Upper Body* move to both sides (left then right) to complete the treatment of the posterior upper body. As lymph drainage watersheds flow, this upper shoulder section follows its own drainage pathway, different than the pattern for the back of shoulders and arms.

Another example of this section-by-section, logical method of application is for the lower body. When addressing the lower extremities (*Step 3* and *Step 5*), be sure to treat one entire leg before going to the other leg.

FOLLOW THE INSTRUCTIONS FOR EACH STEP IN ORDER.

For example, this is the order in which you complete *Step 2: The Back of the Upper Body*.

➤ *Stimulating the Axillary Lymph Nodes* (left)

➤ *The Upper Back* (left)

➤ *The Upper Arms* (left)

➤ *Stimulating the Axillary Lymph Nodes* (right)

➤ *The Upper Back* (right)

➤ *The Upper Arms* (right)

➤ *Finishing the Back of the Upper Body* (left)

➤ *Finishing the Back of the Upper Body* (right)

EXCEPTIONS

For every step of the treatment process, you will find some exceptions plus a few cup-free recommendations to address exceptions as needed. You will find brief notes in each step for any of these instances, but for more detailed information about these exceptional items, please review *Chapter 5: Before Beginning Cupping.*

USING THIS BOOK WHILE YOU WORK

The best way to use this book is to work alongside each page you are on, one step at a time. There are step-by-step instructions, including starting points, line(s) of movement, end points and the recommended treatment process. Also included are Cellulite Focus Options, exceptions, any cup-free recommendations, safety point reminders, anatomy tidbits, and other helpful suggestions wherever applicable.

At the end of this chapter is a *Body-Cupping Map* that lays out the entire treatment process on one page, in one photo with overlays to show each step. This image is useful both as a summary and as a one-page treatment guide. Once you get familiar with the entire treatment process, you will be able to use this one-page map to follow along with as needed. The charted instructions for each of the six steps will guide you through the sequence—no page turning necessary.

In general treatment settings, you will be working standing alongside the recipient's body as they lie on a treatment table. That is how the images in this book appear, from the practitioner's perspective. If you prefer to position yourself otherwise (for example, sitting on a stool), please adjust accordingly, keeping the vantage point of this book in mind.

Treatment Photos

The treatment photos in this book have overlays to show the direction of movement and techniques to be used.

- The star marked on all cupping photos indicates the starting point(s).

- Where there are arrows (any line of movement), that means you can use lift-and-release or moving cups. The arrows point in the direction of the line(s) of movement.

- The Morse Code of Cups photo (on page 55) shows how lift-and-release and moving cups can be combined; this goes for any line of movement, anywhere on the body.

- A few cupping treatment photos (such as the Universal Pass on page 108) have only Xs marked on them. These indicate that this treatment process uses lift-and-release only.

- For the Cup-Free Options (as on page 77), the arrows show the direction in which your fingertips or hands will move.

PREPARING FOR BODY CUPPING

While it is not required, I recommend clean skin for this treatment. That does not mean your clients must shower or be cleansed before this treatment, but not having environmental dirt or excess sweat is best for optimal results. Even though you will be applying oil to do the cupping, it could get messy on the dirt- or sweat-covered skin and, depending on what is covering the skin, whether it be dirt or sunscreen, it can become difficult to clean off the cups. Some people even see brown or gray residues when they use cups over dirty skin.

And considering how open the pores will be after such a treatment, having somewhat cleaner skin will allow for applied products to be absorbed more efficiently; see *Chapter 11: After a Body-Cupping Treatment* for after-care recommendations.

Option: If accessible, saunas, steam rooms or hot tubs are great suggestions. The moist heat will soften the skin, relax the muscles and serve as great preparation for sliding cups across the skin with ease. If you do not have access to these hydrotherapies, steam towel applications or warm compresses will provide similar soft tissue preparation.

OTHER BODY TREATMENTS AND CUPPING

If you are a practitioner who uses other therapeutic tools (such as scrapers, cellulite or adhesion-reducing devices, etc.), there are a few options for you to consider before you combine cupping with other body treatments. You do not want to overwork the body tissues.

Similarly, if you use needles (acupuncture), microneedling or other treatments that break the skin, you will want to be sure to do the body cupping first.

For recommendations, see *Other Treatments and Cupping* on page 88.

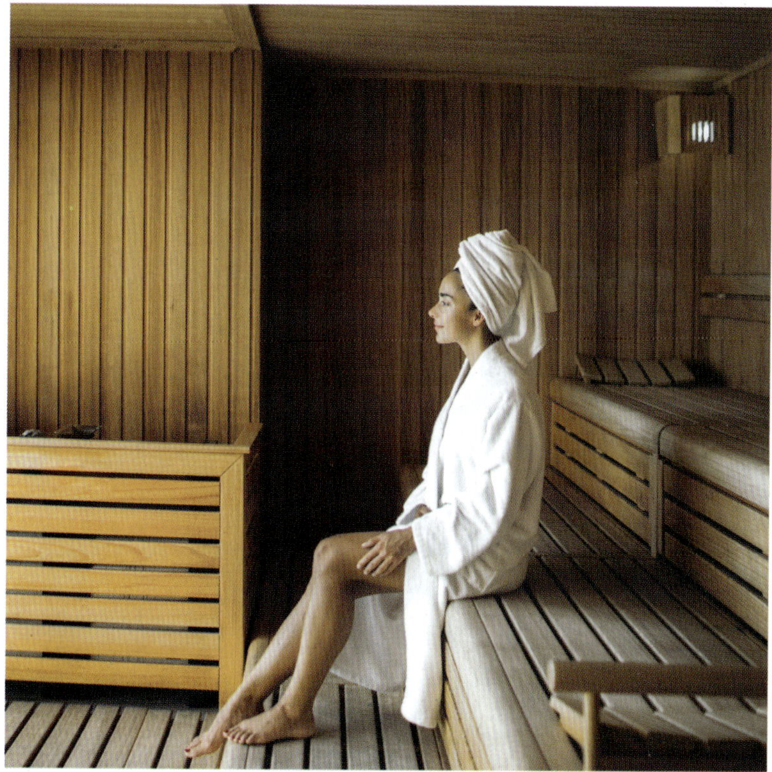

CELLULITE FOCUS OPTIONS

This entire treatment follows lymph drainage pathways. Following this method of application is the best way to safely move cups across the entire body. Doing this treatment without any particular focus areas will still yield nice, smoothing effects on the surface tissues. Since, however, areas of congested cellulite need a little more attention—and this is a cellulite-reduction, focused treatment—there are focus options available for every part of the body.

When choosing to focus on any area, there is a basic principle you must understand. *First* initiate the lymph drainage, *then* focus on the cellulite area and *then* repeat the initial draining movements.

Why? To begin with, the long, draining strokes get the lymph and blood moving, which not only starts the draining process but also warms up the area in preparation for the vigorous, focused movements that come immediately after. The focus area won't be as sensitive and the soft tissues will be more pliable than if starting without those initial lines of movement. Once finished with the focusing moves, repeating the lymph-moving lines of movement will further enhance the drainage and allow for smooth, contouring moves along each line of movement.

While moving cups and lift-and-release are the best techniques for this entire treatment, there are a few more options available for any area of focus. At every Cellulite Focus Option, these additional methods of application (described below) are noted if applicable.

Vigorous moving cups. This method of application is the most popular with cupping for cellulite. Using light pressure as you would with the lymph draining lines of movement, apply moving cups in a fast-paced yet comfortable manner. This will really stir up the congested area, breaking down the superficial adhesions of cellulite. At each focus location, the best direction of movement in which to apply these fast-moving cups is described.

Focus cupping on stubborn divots. This is where some more specific cupping can be applied. While the entire body-cupping treatment uses lift-and-release or moving cups, any

CELLULITE SHORTCUTS

While the best results will come from the full body treatment sequence, there are a few shortcuts available if desired, for self-care or quick client spot focuses. See page 237 at the end of this chapter for *Quick-Fix Cellulite Shortcuts*.

stubborn adhesions can be cupped in a more focused manner if needed. (See the optional methods of application for spot focus, below.) Since these are less common methods of application, at every focus option you will find an instruction to "apply additional focused cellulite cupping as needed," and a reference back to this section for further information on options to choose. Just as using the Morse Code of Cups becomes a natural way to use cups across any surface, you will find that you naturally choose to incorporate these specific methods of cellulite focus into the treatment wherever necessary.

Optional Methods of Application for Focus on Stubborn Cellulite Dimples

- **Repetitive lift-and-release.** Deep cellulite dimples indicate severe restriction, which may be sensitive to anything too focused. Repeatedly applying lift-and-release over any of these sites will help to jostle things loose. With time and perhaps several treatments, this will yield results that allow for more vigorous or focused cupping without discomfort.

- **Twisting the cup.** Just as twisting a cup helps release wrinkles, using moving cups over sites of cellulite while you twist the cup will help loosen the restrictions across the region. When done in this manner, the sensation is comparable to kneading done with hands.

- **Stationary cup—but for less than three minutes!** In extreme cases, a stationary cup can be applied to really focus on the depth of restrictions. This technique is the most common method of cupping (known for other cupping applications), but it can potentially yield cupping marks and is not recommended for anyone very sensitive to cupping. Be sure to limit the length of time any one cup is applied. Because cups pull fluids into tissues, prolonged stationary cups can create surface fluid stagnation, which will have to be drained from the area. Limit stationary cups to less than three minutes at any location.

Regardless of the technique you choose or the technique that is suggested, your goal is to focus on cellulite in a way that is best for the recipient. If you find one method works well for one person and a different method works for another, go for it!

As long as the person you are treating isn't feeling discomfort and you do not see the area getting visibly overstimulated (very red and puffy), you can feel confident that the techniques and methods of application described here will yield benefits.

TREATMENT POINTERS

OPTIMAL SUCTION PRESSURE

There is no need to use strong suction pressure to address the stagnation of lymph, adipose cells and sticky fascia, given their shallow depth. Using lighter suction pressure to address any focus areas is best; it will do so without damaging the soft tissues, blood vessels or nerves.

There are many other modalities that address cellulite in a very aggressive—and often painful—manner. They work *into* these micro-adhesions to break them up; at times this can be a necessary evil to make such work effective.

Cups, however, work with negative pressure. Applying them over an area of cellulite should be less about strong suction and more about using the cups skillfully. There is no reason for a painful treatment. Instead, it should feel invigorating and energizing.

While each of the treatment pointers listed here is discussed elsewhere in this book, they are included here for quick reference as you work through the body-cupping treatment process.

- **Cups should be larger in size.** Use the largest cup you can to comfortably treat every body part. The larger cups should be used over larger body parts (gluteal region, midsection), and relative to the body part being treated (gluteal region compared to the upper arm).
- **Use moving cups or lift-and-release techniques—no stationary cups.** The intention with this treatment is to improve circulation. Regardless of which technique is used, be sure to keep it active. Use either technique to address the tissue accordingly or combine the two as necessary (known as the Morse Code of Cups—see page 55). *Exception:* Any cellulite focus areas will have the option for brief stationary cup placement over stubborn cellulite dimples. This is the only exception for using stationary cups.
- **Suction pressure should be lighter.** Cupping the surfaces of the body for cellulite or body contouring follows the natural flow of lymph; lighter suction pressure will more effectively address the superficial anatomy where lymph drainage pathways exist.
- **Be aware of the pace of application.** Movements should be slower for draining and faster for cellulite focus. Regardless of the pace, make it a rhythmic application. Remember, the entire body treatment should take no more than one hour. To review the benefits of these varied paces, see page 58 in *Chapter 3: How to Use Cups.*

Choosing Cupping Sets

While it does not matter which cupping set you use, I personally recommend using a manual pump cup set to control the lighter suction pressure required for most of this treatment. However, for cellulite focus areas, I recommend using silicone squeeze cups, so one hand can stabilize the body part and the other can work with the more vigorous movements. The photographs for each step show the recommended cupping set where necessary.

- **Follow the step-by-step instructions as they are given.** This will ensure safe and effective natural circulation of blood and lymph. On page 174 is a basic map of the lymph drainage pathways. *The Body-Cupping Map* on page 235 shows each step and indicates the direction in which it should be worked. Also, there will be some steps where you begin that region by stimulating lymph nodes. Addressing these collection areas to "unclog the drain" before you move fluids there is necessary for proper sequencing of lymph drainage.
- **Remember repetitive movements.** Three to five passes are recommended over every line of movement for a universal treatment. When focusing on an area, you may do up to ten or twenty stimulating passes, then repeat the three to five slower, draining passes over the area before you move on to the next section.

Note: *If you have questions about cupping for lymph drainage before you begin the treatment, review Chapters 1 and 2.*

Still have questions? Consider contacting a certified therapeutic cupping practitioner or a manual lymph drainage therapist for more insight about the lymphatic system, this type of cupping treatment or perhaps to experience a treatment first-hand for yourself.

CUPPING 101

COMFORTABLE MOVING CUPS

Be sure to switch to the lift-and-release technique for any location where a moving cup is uncomfortable or difficult to use, such as over the shoulder blades, any "stuck" area of soft tissue or along the extremities if any location is sensitive. You may choose to mix moving cups and lift-and-release at any time (see the Morse Code of Cups on page 55).

Some people receiving cupping therapy for the first time may be more sensitive to initial applications, as the body is not familiar with the concept of negative-pressure therapies. You may choose to incorporate the lift-and-release technique wherever needed to ensure a more comfortable and effective experience.

STEP-BY-STEP BODY CUPPING

Preliminary Steps

There are two preliminary steps that are almost always done before beginning the six steps of the body-cupping treatment. These two steps don't use cups but will help prepare your client's body for cupping for lymph drainage.

First, offering an abdominal massage is a great way to stimulate the body's lymphatic activities. Next, manual stimulation of the supraclavicular lymph nodes and terminal thoracic ducts is a must in most lymph drainage treatments.

OPTIONAL BUT RECOMMENDED

While neither of these two preliminary steps is required, they are highly recommended for anyone who wants the most benefits from this treatment. The occasions to consider not taking these preliminary steps are if the client received bodywork earlier that day, or possibly the day before, since their body will already have been stimulated.

Alternatively, many cellulite treatments omit these steps without issue; however, in my professional opinion (and that of most manual lymph drainage therapists), including these two quick opening moves guarantees an even more effective treatment for lymph movement.

Once you have completed these preliminary steps, you are ready to begin *Step 1: The Middle and Lower Back*.

ADDRESS THE ABDOMEN MANUALLY

In manual lymph drainage therapy, before a session begins, the therapist typically administers abdominal massage and encourages deep belly breathing to stimulate the concentration of lymphatic activity in this region. Alternatively, simply massaging the abdomen with comfortable pressure in a clockwise manner, following the direction of the large intestine, will stimulate the abdomen.

This is the first preliminary step. While not required, I strongly recommend this abdominal massage before body cupping, since it addresses the core of the body where a lot of supporting systemic activity takes place.

Given the focus on lymphatic movement in this treatment, addressing the abdominal area is a great place to start for many people. There is a wealth of lymphatic activity in the midsection of the body, so choosing to gently manipulate the abdomen before beginning body-cupping treatment will further "unclog the drain" to encourage the lymph to easily flow.

Assess the state of the abdominal area, which is the most central region of the body. If the person being treated suffers from excessive abdominal congestion, such as constipation, treating the abdominal area first is a good choice.

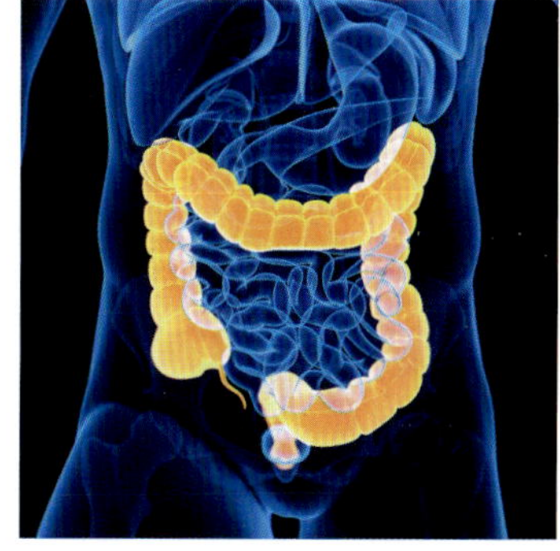

When massaging the abdomen, you follow the large intestine (highlighted) in a clockwise direction.

STIMULATE THE UPPER BODY FOR LYMPH DRAINAGE

This is the second preliminary step. Before we begin the body treatment, it is important to stimulate the supraclavicular lymph nodes and, indirectly, the thoracic ducts.

Stimulating the most powerful lymph nodes of the entire body further "unclogs the drain."

There are two possible areas you can stimulate for the upper body—the primary location is below the anterior triangle area and the second, optional location is the axilla or axillary space, here called the axilla armpit.

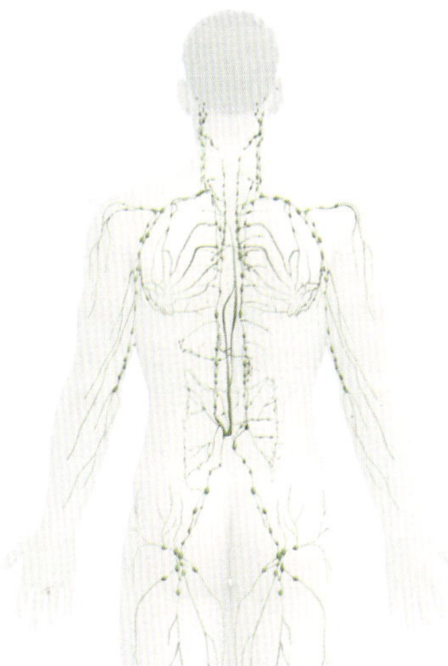

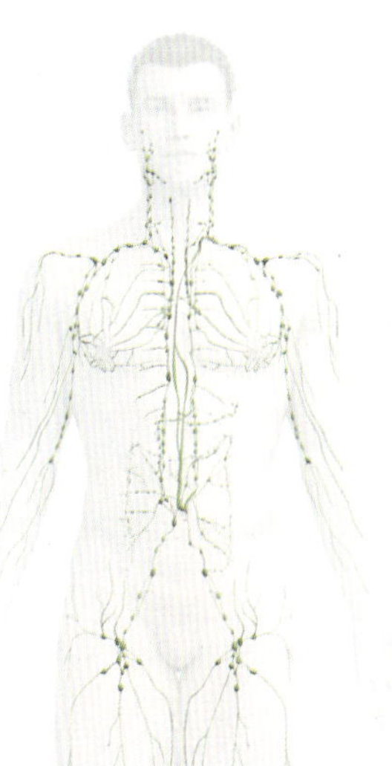

For more about the lymphatic system, see page 30 in *Chapter 1: The Science of How Cupping Affect the Body*. To refresh your knowledge of lymph watersheds and pathways, see page 174 in *Chapter 9: Body Cupping for Cellulite and Contouring*.

Address the Abdomen Manually

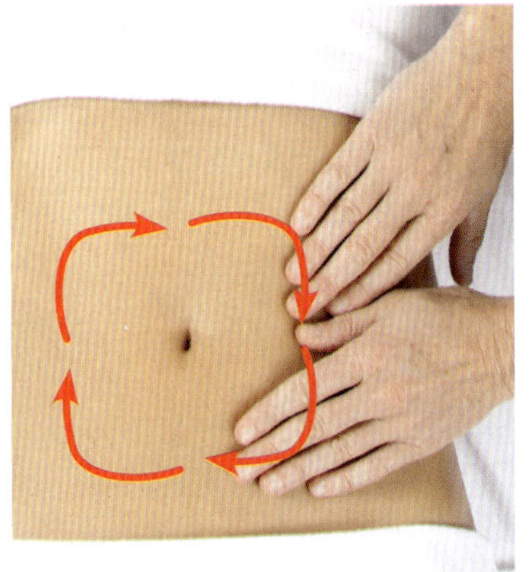

Gently massage the abdomen in a clockwise, circular direction.

I strongly recommend this abdominal massage before body cupping, since it addresses the core of the body where a lot of supporting systemic activity takes place.

For this step, your client is lying on their back, arms relaxed and at their sides on the table. You will massage the abdomen with comfortable pressure in a clockwise direction, following the direction of the large intestine. Adding this optional opening treatment will promote lymphatic activity before the client turns over onto their stomach and the cupping treatment begins.

LOCATION

To best follow the flow of the large intestine, this location covers the majority of the abdominal space; from the tops of the anterior superior iliac spine (the ASIS) and the front hip bones to the bottom of the rib cage and circling the navel.

TREATMENT PROCESS

➤ *Always travel in a clockwise direction when doing abdominal massage.* This is the natural direction of movement within this part of the digestive system.

➤ Begin applying circles on the person's left side, starting in the upper left quadrant of their midsection. Starting here will gently clear the descending colon first, which is the most proximal part of the large intestines.

➤ Begin to makes large circles, moving clockwise around the client's abdomen.

➤ From the upper left quadrant, move hands down toward their left ASIS, then travel under the navel and across toward their right ASIS, then up toward the right lower rib cage (in their right upper quadrant), then travel above the navel and across to their left lower rib cage where the circle began.

➤ Repeat this circular massaging five to twenty times; the more congested the region is, the more circular movements are recommended.

Once finished, continue to the other optional opening move (*Stimulating the Upper Body for Lymph Drainage*) or instruct the client to turn over (prone) and begin the cupping treatment.

Stimulate the Upper Body for Lymph Drainage

ANTERIOR TRIANGLE AREA

This cup-free application is easiest to do before you pick up the cups and just before you apply the lubricant.

Begin with the person receiving treatment in the prone (face-down) position, arms relaxed and extended off the sides of the table or alongside their body if that is comfortable for them.

For this step, you are standing at the head of your client, using both hands to treat both sides at the same time. In this starting position, your fingertips will be within the lower anterior triangle space, so be sure to use very light pressure only.

LOCATION

This area is just inside the collarbones, on each side of the throat. Your fingertips will just contact the clavicle collarbones, resting lightly within the anterior triangle.

TREATMENT PROCESS

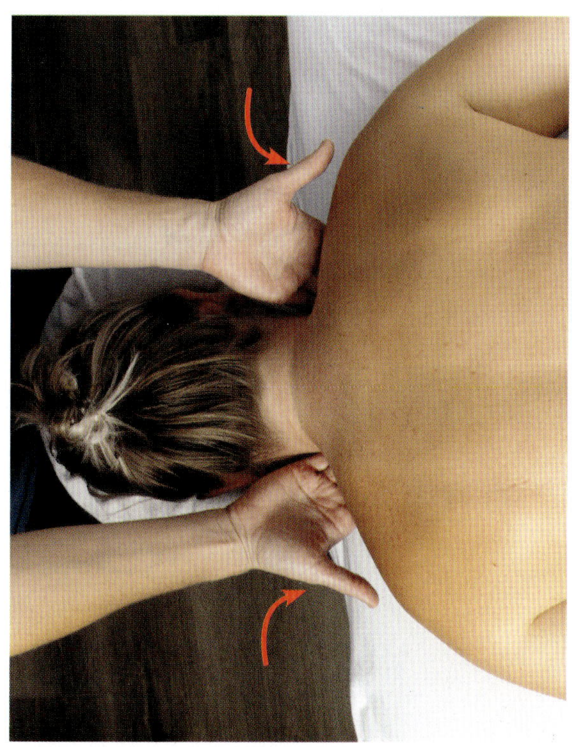

➤ Place relaxed but flattened fingers just above the clavicle collarbones, in the front of the neck space as viewed from this position (see the photo). I say "relaxed but flattened" because the fingers are not rigid or digging into the skin, but instead relaxed, flattened and resting on the skin's surface for a very light lymph-stimulating move.

➤ Gently pump your fingertips into the body in a small, skin-stretching circle up and forward toward the clavicle. The circles are very small, barely stretching the skin.

➤ Repeat these small, pumping circles three to five times.

Stimulate the Upper Body for Lymph Drainage

AXILLARY LYMPH NODE REGION

If there is excessive congestion in the upper body, consider stimulating the axillary armpit area lymph nodes, too. An indication that this option would be beneficial is if the client showed engorged or puffy skin around the bra strap area, which is a common site of soft tissue congestion (see photo, bottom left).

LOCATION
The area to be treated is in the axilla armpit.

TREATMENT PROCESS
➤ Rest relaxed but flattened fingers in the armpit region.
➤ Gently flex all the fingers into the armpit and out again, making a small, pumping motion into the body and out again. I often describe this motion as if you are telling the lymph to "come here" by the way you bend and straighten your fingers into the armpit.
➤ Note that these circles are not meant to dig into the armpit. Rather, they should gently press into the skin to stimulate the regional lymph nodes located just under the skin's surface.
➤ Repeat these gentle, skin-pressing circles three to five times in each axilla armpit.
➤ Continue to *Step 1: The Middle and Lower Back.*

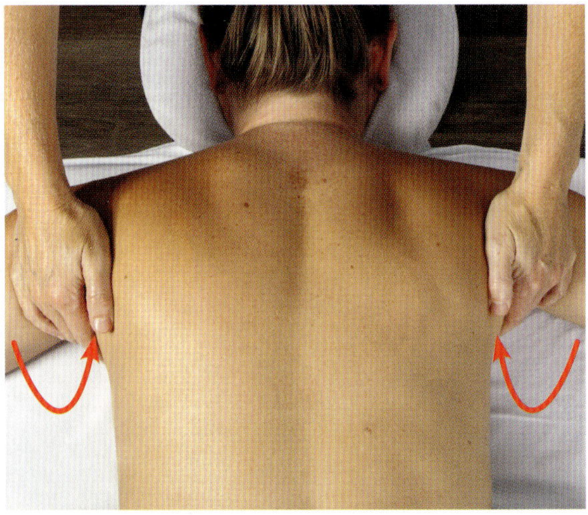

An example of excessive congestion near posterior axillary space

The Middle and Lower Back

As part of the body's core, the middle and lower back are considered "the back of the abdomen." This area measures from just below the shoulder blades in the mid-thoracic region down to the posterior iliac crest of the hip bones. This is a common region for lymphatic congestion because of various factors, from hip tension or low back pains, to clothing restrictions or a sedentary lifestyle. Whether addressing cellulite, "love handles" or "muffin top," contouring treatments often focus on this region.

The paths of lymph drainage travel around the sides of the body, draining into the lower abdomen. Since the person being treated is lying on their stomach (which makes it impossible to finish the total line of movement to its end point), the lines of movement will end at "drop-off" locations along the sides of the body. Then, when the client is supine, the lines of movement will be "picked up," continuing onto the lower abdomen to complete the drainage.

WHY CUP THE MIDDLE AND LOWER BACK?

Cupping through the middle and lower back is incredibly therapeutic for lymph drainage. The lift offered by cupping helps to decompress any "stuck" areas (such as impressions from compression garments), and it feels great. With every pass of the cup, a comforting yet sculpting sensation is palpable across this curvy anatomy. Cupping in this region also relieves low back tension, as the cups move from the low back toward the side of the body, along a common "belt line" of tension.

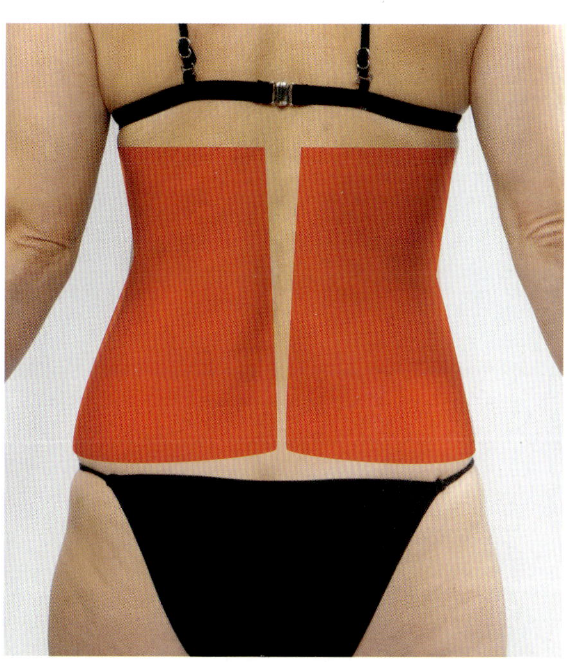

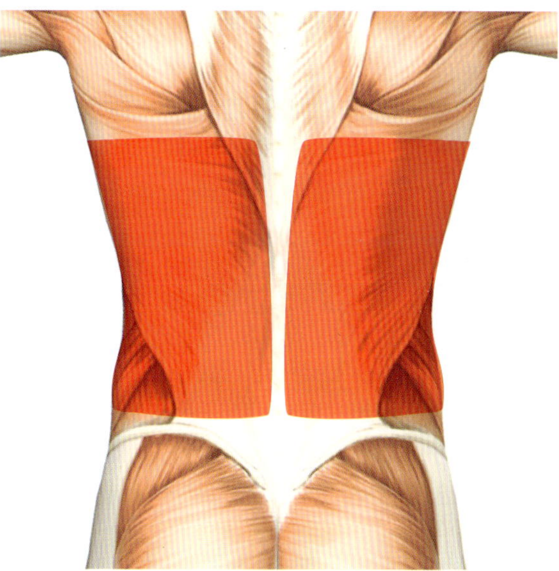

The Middle and Lower Back

LOCATION

This area covers the low back and posterior midsection, from the hip bone (posterior iliac crest) up to the mid-thoracic lower rib cage section. While every body is different, three lines of movement with a larger cup will usually address this entire region.

STARTING POINT

Each starting point is at the side of the lower spine, the first beginning just above the hip bones.

LINE OF MOVEMENT

Follow along the hip bone, progressing out toward the side of the body.

END POINT

Each end point is at the side of the body.

Since the end point for this section of lymph drainage is in the lower abdomen, consider the side of the body a "drop-off" location, where you will "pick up" the lymph and continue to the lower abdomen after the person has turned over.

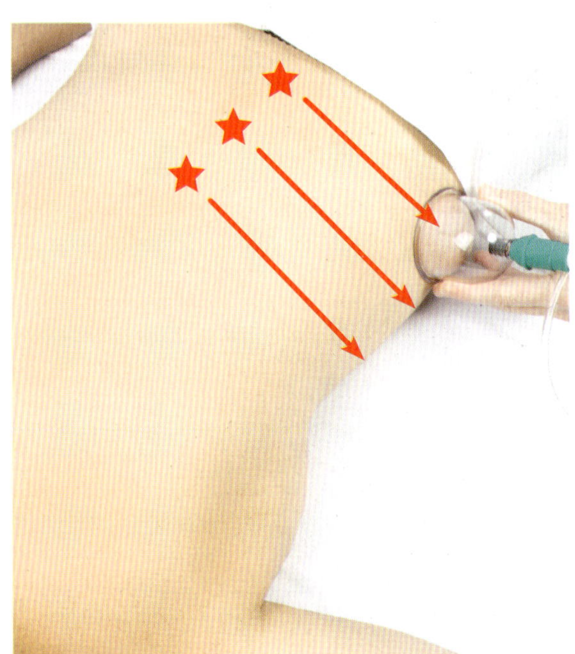

TREATMENT PROCESS

➤ Attach the cup at the starting point and follow the line of movement using moving cups and/or lift-and-release to the end point. Detach the cup and return to the starting point.

➤ Repeat each line of movement three to five times.

➤ Progress your way up to the bottom of the shoulder blade, one cup-width at a time. In all, a total of about nine to fifteen passes to cover the entire section.

➤ Repeat this sequence on the right side of the body.

➤ Once this section is complete, continue to *Step 2: The Back of the Upper Body.*

If choosing to add in the Cellulite Focus Option, proceed with that option before continuing on to *Step 2.*

The Middle and Lower Back

CELLULITE FOCUS OPTION

This section of the body, where we find what we lovingly refer to as "love handles" or "muffin top," is a common site for cellulite and lymphatic congestion. After you work on the posterior midsection, you can add some stimulating side-to-side movements to focus on the cellulite and contouring.

Use faster, vigorous movements to focus on this region.

Stubborn cellulite dimples? Apply additional focused cellulite cupping as needed. Refer to page 182 for more details on these advanced methods of application.

TREATMENT PROCESS

➤ With the same lighter suction pressure, follow the same lines of movements with side-to-side movements (see photo) at a faster yet comfortable pace.

➤ Repeat these fast-paced, side-to-side movements five to ten times.

➤ Cover each line of movement in this section in this similar manner.

➤ Once finished, repeat a few passes with the original, slower-paced draining lines of movement from starting point to end point.

➤ Repeat this optional sequence on the right side of the body before moving on to *Step 2: The Back of the Upper Body.*

➤ Once this section is complete, continue to *Step 2: The Back of the Upper Body.*

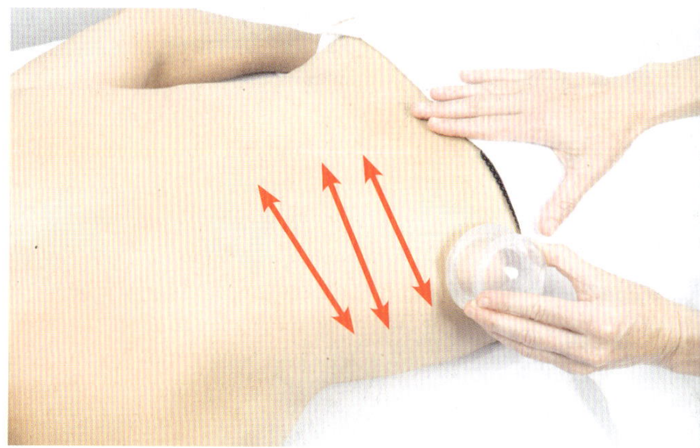

CUPPING MARK POTENTIAL

Remember, any Cellulite Focus Option suggested in this book has the potential for minor cupping marks, so be sure to visually monitor the tissue as you work.

Comfort and Safety

The person being treated should feel no discomfort or ripping or tearing sensations when receiving this more vigorous application. While this style of cupping is meant to be stimulating, it should never be painful. Always check lubrication, suction pressure and the comfort of your client when choosing to add in these optional, advanced techniques.

The Back of the Upper Body

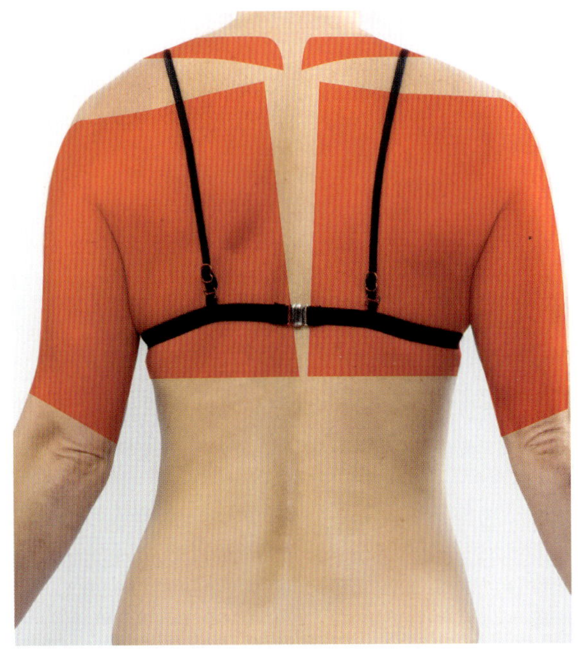

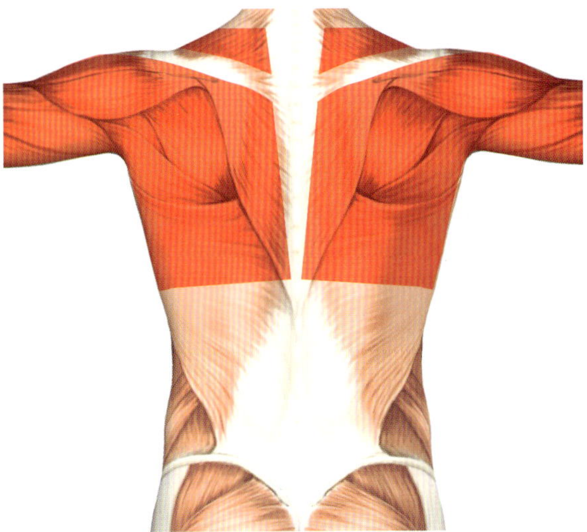

Continuing up the torso, this area covers the upper back and upper arms, from the mid-back, where *Step 1* ended, to the top of the shoulder blades and out to the elbows. This is often an area of lymphatic congestion and cosmetic focus. Some people have congestion due to clothing restrictions (such as bras) or they want to focus on the "winged" backs of the arms.

This entire region drains into the axillary armpit area, where the average adult has twenty to forty lymph nodes. For this reason, it is necessary to stimulate the regional lymph nodes before you bring fluids into the region.

WHY CUP ACROSS THE BACK OF THE UPPER BODY?

Cupping through this area supports the overall lymph drainage process, contours the back of arms and upper back and provides muscular relief throughout this often-tense region. Your client remains in the prone position for this step.

For greatest benefit, we divide this region into four parts: *Stimulating the Axillary Lymph Nodes, The Upper Back, The Upper Arms,* and *Finishing the Back of the Upper Body.* You will complete the first three parts of this sequence first on the left and then on the right. *Finishing the Back of the Upper Body* is done after you have completed these three parts on both sides; you are literally finishing the back of the upper body section entirely.

Stimulating the Axillary Lymph Nodes is necessary as part of the general lymphatic sequencing. Before treating the rest of the upper body, applying a few gentle applications of lift-and-release will stimulate all the lymph nodes located in this region to receive lymph from the surrounding areas. Since this is within an endangerment site, cupping is very light, using barely any suction at all. This step "unclogs the drain" to prepare the upper body region so it will drain into the axilla. There is a Cup-Free Option for this part of *Step 2,* since you are working directly in an endangerment site.

The Upper Back is not a common site for cellulite, but there may be lymphatic stagnation present, most obviously as skin that hangs over bra straps or shows looseness near the back of the armpit. Whether it is an area of concern or not, it is still important to address since it is part of the total lymphatic sequence.

The Upper Arms are also important to address, both cosmetically and lymphatically. This is often an area where cellulite treatments are of benefit. Also, the upper arms can reflect general tension patterns connected to the shoulders. Note that the back of the arms can be very sensitive if there is a lot of fluid or muscle tension, so I recommend using lift-and-release or the combination Morse Code of Cups here. There is also a Cellulite Focus Option for this part.

Finishing the Back of the Upper Body is a multi-purpose closing move for the entire upper body. First, it addresses the topmost parts of the shoulders, which are not treated in *The Upper Back.* This area is very small, but lymph here flows forward over the tops of shoulders, not out toward the axilla. Cupping through this small area can relieve potential fluid retention as well as common muscle tension patterns. Also, this revisits the supraclavicular lymph nodes and thoracic duct region, where the entire treatment began. As with the Universal Pass in the face-cupping treatment, this quick step is necessary to keep lymph fluids moving along the drainage pathways.

POSSIBLE REPEAT STIMULATION AREA

In *Stimulating the Axillary Lymph Nodes* (see page 196), you revisit the same location you may have stimulated earlier. It was recommended as a pre-treatment option (see page 190) especially helpful if your client has excessive lymphatic congestion in this area, usually due to bra strap restrictions. Yes, it is necessary to repeat the stimulation here even if already done as a preliminary step before *Step 1* of the treatment.

Stimulating the Axillary Lymph Nodes

Begin stimulating these regional lymph nodes by working directly in the armpit endangerment site with very light suction pressure.

LOCATION
This treatment area occurs in the soft tissue space of the armpit.

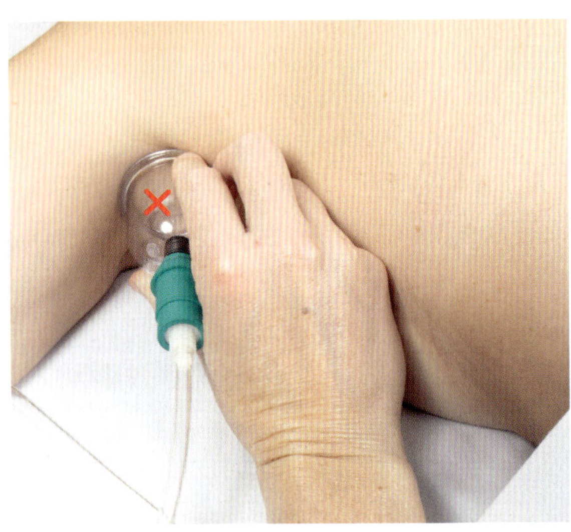

TREATMENT PROCESS
➤ Lightly apply the lift-and-release technique three to five times in the exact same location. Think of this as a gentle, therapeutic plunger.
➤ Once one axilla has been stimulated, continue to the next part of *Step 2, The Upper Back*.

Note: *Because this is an endangerment site, the suction should barely lift the skin.*

Stimulating the Axillary Lymph Nodes

CUP-FREE OPTION

If the cups will not work for whatever reason in this region (for example, excessive body hair) or if you prefer not to use a cup in this area, follow the Cup-Free Option, which mimics a manual lymph drainage treatment technique. If standing at the head of the table, consider stimulating both axillary lymph nodes at the same time, using both hands (one hand in each axillary space). If not, follow the instructions to one axilla, then stimulate the other.

TREATMENT PROCESS

Using the same location as instructed with a cup, use your relaxed but flattened fingers to create small inward-pumping circles into the axilla.

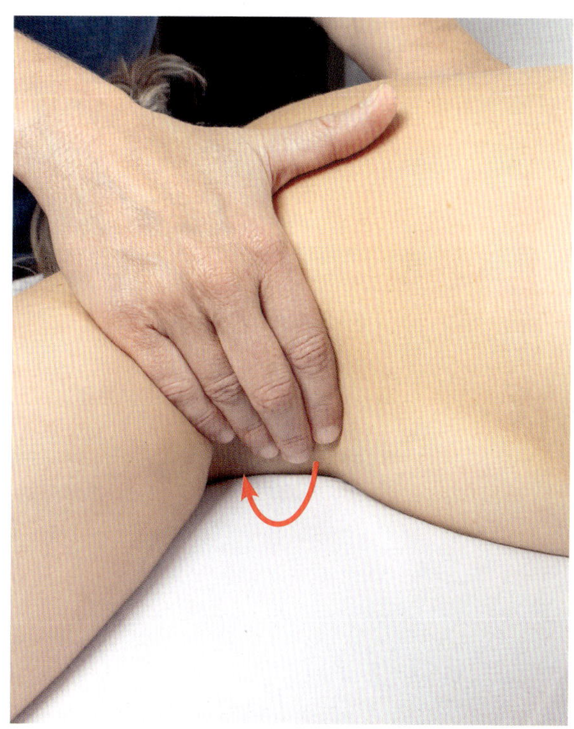

➤ Rest relaxed but flattened fingers at the armpit region, and gently flex the fingers *into* the armpit and out again, making a small, gentle circle into the body and out again.

Note: *These circles are not meant to dig into the armpit. Rather, they should gently press into the skin to stimulate the regional lymph nodes located just under the skin's surface.*

➤ Repeat these gentle, skin-pressing circles three to five times in each location.
➤ Once this section is completed, proceed to the next part of *Step 2, The Upper Back*.

The Upper Back

Begin addressing the upper back at the bottom of the shoulders, where *Step 1* ended, just below the shoulder blade.

Consider the axilla end point a "drop-off" location for the upper body.

LOCATION
This area is from the mid-back up to the top of the shoulder blades, and from the spine to the armpits (on both sides).

STARTING POINT
Start along the side of the spine, in line with the bottom of the shoulder blade.

LINE OF MOVEMENT
You will move from the midline of the body out to the side, toward the axilla (armpit). As you work upward, the lines of movement will travel directly over the shoulder blades, angling toward the axilla.

END POINT
At the side of the body, along the outside edge of the shoulder blade where the axilla begins. This is just outside the armpit, where the axillary lymph nodes were previously stimulated; consider this a "drop-off" location for the upper body.

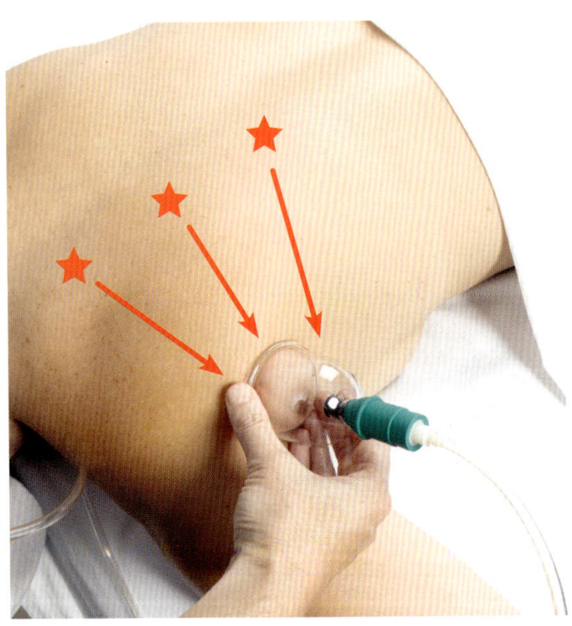

TREATMENT PROCESS
- Attach the cup at the starting point(s) and follow the line(s) of movement using moving cups and/or lift-and-release to the end point. Detach the cup and return to the starting point.
- Repeat each line of movement three to five times.
- One cup-width at a time, progress your way across the shoulder region, working out toward the axilla end point every time.
- Once this section is completed, proceed to the next part of *Step 2, The Upper Arms.*

Note: *If you cannot slide the cup over the shoulder blade comfortably, use the lift-and-release technique to move across it.*

The Upper Arms

Begin addressing the upper arms near the elbow. I recommend you position your client's arm over the side of the table, bent and relaxed (see photo). However, if this is uncomfortable, the arm can remain alongside their body on the table; just be sure to work along the triceps muscle and not along the more sensitive inside line of upper arm.

LOCATION

The area being cupped is the backside of the upper arm, from the elbow to the back outer edge of shoulder blade.

STARTING POINT

Start just above the elbow.

LINE OF MOVEMENT

Move along the back of the upper arm, progressing toward the back of the armpit area.

END POINT

End at the drop-off location at the outer edge of the armpit; the same end point as *The Upper Back*.

TREATMENT PROCESS

➤ Attach the cup at the starting point and follow the line of movement using moving cups and/or lift-and-release to the end point. Detach the cup and return to the starting point.
➤ Repeat this line of movement three to five times.
➤ The average upper arm will accommodate one or two lines of movement; in all, there will be an average of six to ten passes here.
➤ Repeat this sequence on the right side.
➤ Once this section is completed, proceed to the final part of *Step 2, Finishing the Back of the Upper Body*.

If choosing to add in the Cellulite Focus Option, proceed with that option before restarting *Step 2* on the other side of the body.

FAQ

WHAT ABOUT THE INSIDE OF THE UPPER ARM?

While it can be cupped, too, there are many lymph nodes, nerves and blood vessels more superficially exposed here. So, if choosing to cup along this line, do so with very light suction pressure for moving cups, or simply use the lift-and-release from the inside of the elbow up toward the axilla.

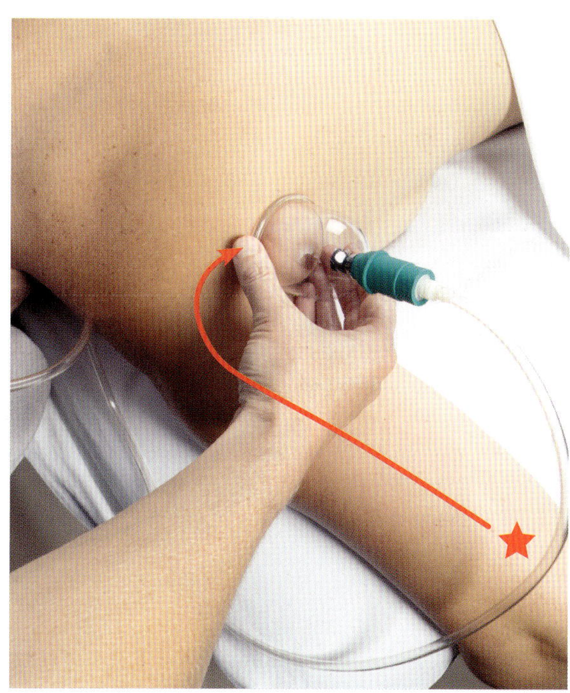

The Upper Arms

CELLULITE FOCUS OPTION

Sometimes referred to as "wings," the flesh at the back of the upper arms is a common site for cellulite. Especially if a bra strap causes constriction, there can be fluid retention here, contributing to unsightly cellulite dimples.

After finishing the treatment process on page 199, use faster, vigorous movements to focus on cellulite in this region.

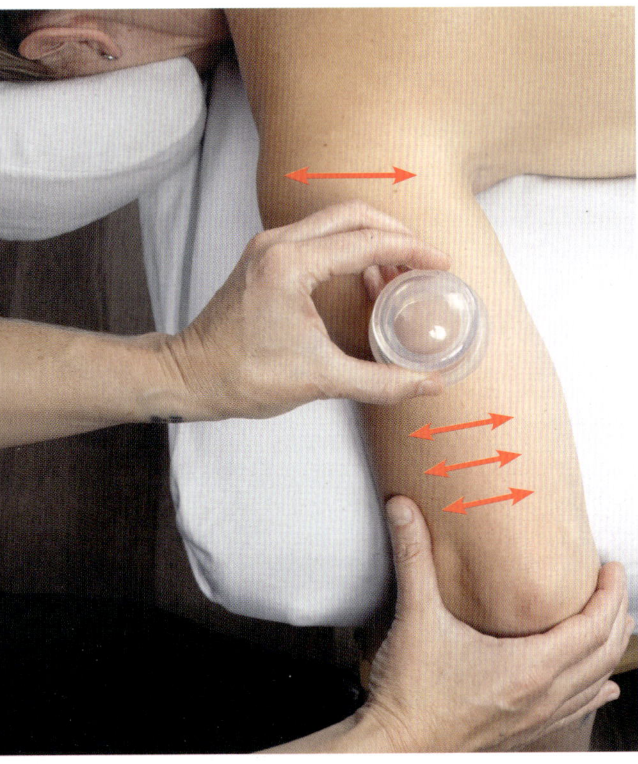

Stubborn cellulite dimples? Apply additional focused cellulite cupping as needed. Refer to page 182 at the beginning of this chapter for more details on these advanced methods of application.

TREATMENT PROCESS

➤ With the same lighter suction pressure, move the cup side to side across the back of the upper arm at a faster yet comfortable pace.

Note: *Do not go up and down the arm (from armpit to elbow), as that can be more sensitive than side-to-side. Moving up and down the arm inevitably goes against the natural flow of lymph (if you move toward the elbow), which can feel odd to many people.*

➤ Repeat these fast-paced, side-to-side movements five to ten times, traveling from elbow to shoulder and back down again.

Suggestion: *Use one hand to anchor the arm around the elbow area and the other hand to manipulate the cup.* Although this is not required, the recipient's arm may sway and move around if not held in place. Also, consider rotating your hand at the wrist as you do it for your comfort; envision turning a door knob.

➤ Once finished, repeat a few passes with the original, slower-paced draining lines of movement from starting point to end point.
➤ Then, repeat these three parts of *Step 2* on the right side, including this *Cellulite Reduction Option* if desired.
➤ Then continue to the final part of *Step 2, Finishing the Back of the Upper Body.*

Finishing the Back of the Upper Body

This region is very small yet important to address for total lymphatic treatments. This area, called the supraclavicular drainage region, is the uppermost part of the shoulders, and it is above the upper back region that was just treated. There may be lymphatic congestion here, as when a restrictive bra strap digs into the top of the shoulders. This is also a location of much shoulder tension, since it travels over the top of the upper trapezius muscles. Treating this small region at the end of the entire upper body sequence before moving on to the lower body is important, easy and quick to do.

LOCATION

This small area covers the tops of the shoulders, from the spine of the scapula (topmost bony ridge of the shoulder blade), out to the acromioclavicular (AC) joint, where the scapula hooks on to the clavicle, and forward to the clavicles. If you are looking down over the top of the head, it resembles a diamond-shaped area. This space is very short, your hand's-width at most.

STARTING POINT

Start at the top of the scapula, alongside the spine (on the left or right, respectively). See the stars on the photo on the next page.

LINE OF MOVEMENT

Move across the top of the shoulder, forward toward the clavicle.

END POINT

End in the soft tissue space just inside the clavicle. This is the exact same location where the entire treatment began, using your fingertips to stimulate all lymphatic activity.

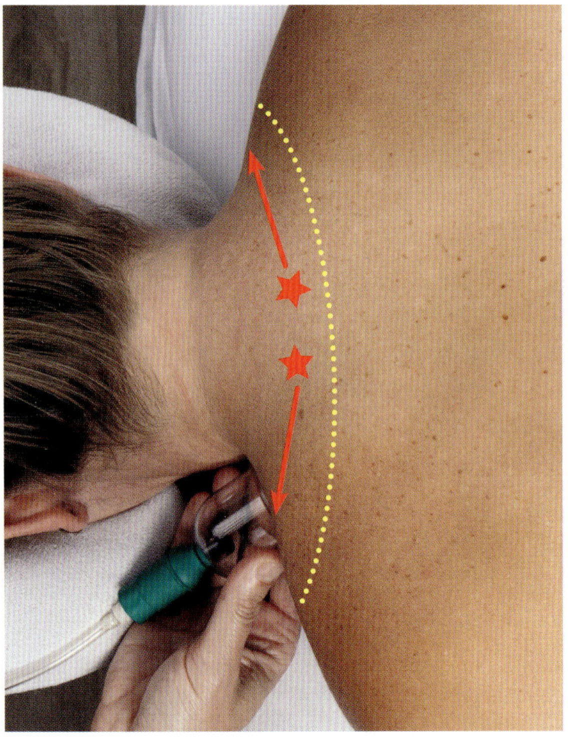

This section is small, quick to do and necessary after you have completed the entire posterior upper body treatment. Use a smaller cup here, or simply use your hands to treat both sides simultaneously before continuing to the next step.

TREATMENT PROCESS

➤ Attach the cup at the starting point and follow the line of movement using moving cups and/or lift-and-release to the end point. Detach the cup and return to the starting point.

➤ Repeat this small line of movement three to five times.

Note: *It may be challenging to use a moving cup here because of the anatomical contour and small space. Use the lift-and-release technique if necessary. Or simply use your hands to follow the same lines of movement for a quick and effective Cup-Free Option.*

➤ Repeat this sequence on the right side of the body.

➤ Once this section is complete, continue to *Step 3: The Back of the Lower Body*, treating one leg first, then the other.

The Back of the Lower Body

Moving into the lower body, we encounter one of the most common areas for cellulite and contouring treatments. The gluteal region includes the buttocks and back side of the hips, which connects into the backs of the thighs.

WHY CUP THE BACK OF THE LOWER BODY?

Because this area experiences compression due to sitting and constriction from clothing, it is a popular site for cupping for cellulite reduction. Muscle tension relief is an added benefit. However, it should be noted that this area can be quite sensitive to cupping, so be sure to work mindfully within each client's comfort levels.

For greatest benefit, we divide this region into three parts: *The Gluteal Region, The Back of the Thighs* and *Stimulating the Popliteal Lymph Nodes.* There is also a *Back of the Lower Leg Option.*

Note: *This treatment addresses the back of one leg entirely before the other.*

The Gluteal Region is important to address cosmetically and lymphatically. It is one of the most common areas for cellulite focus, as well as general tension patterns that connect to the low back, hips and legs. Cellulite here is common since we sit on the buttocks, adding to the compressing of soft tissues here. Clothing can also contribute to congestion here, as waist bands can create restrictions through the midsection, interrupting the drainage of this area forward into the groin area. There is a Cellulite Focus Option for this part.

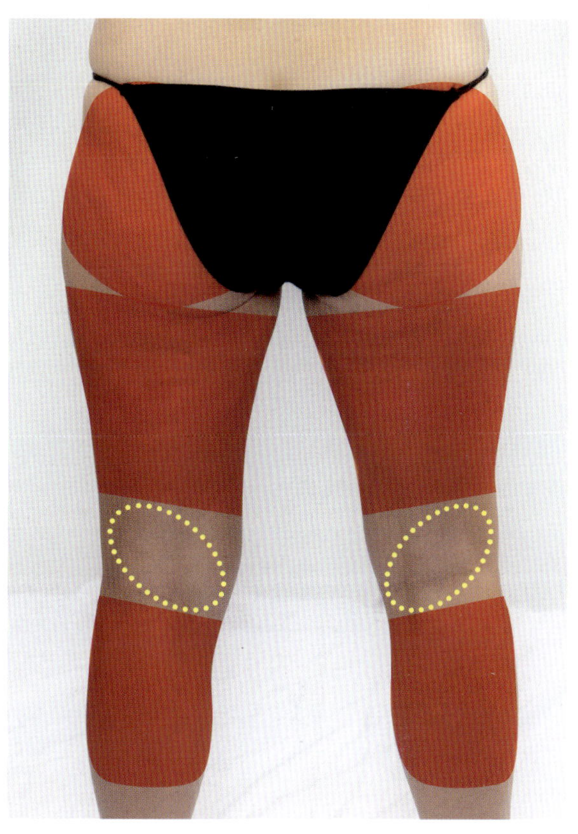

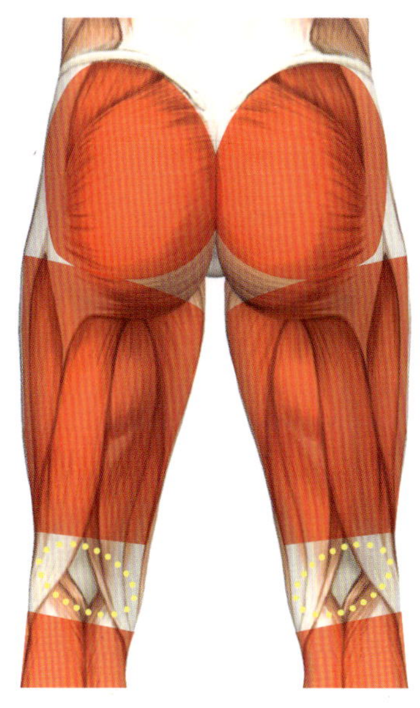

The Back of the Thighs is a continuation of the buttocks. It typically presents with cellulite here if there is some in the gluteal region. Sitting and compression concerns also affect the back of the thighs, which makes this treatment most beneficial when done across the entire region collectively. There is also a Cellulite Focus Option for this part.

Stimulating the Popliteal Lymph Nodes is a vital part of lymph drainage for the legs. There are many lymph nodes here that collect fluids from the lower leg, bringing them up to the groin. Since this is within an endangerment site, very light suction—barely any suction at all—is used here. While most of the work is done above this vulnerable area, quickly and gently stimulating these lymph nodes "unclogs the drain" in the middle of the leg, which is essential for the total leg-draining experience. There is a Cup-Free Option for this final part of *Step 3,* since you are working directly in an endangerment site.

An additional treatment to consider if possible is the *Back of the Lower Leg Option.* While this area is not typically involved with cellulite issues, there may be some circulatory challenges here as well. Choosing the add this distal part of the lower extremity will further support the total lymphatic drainage processes.

The Gluteal Region

The first line of movement for the *Middle and Lower Back* and this line of movement for the *Gluteal Region* share drop-off end point locations. Remember, when the person turns over, face-up, the lymph will be picked up from here and taken to the final end point for regional drainage in the lower abdomen.

LOCATION

The entire buttock is addressed here; from the top of the thigh to the posterior iliac crest of the hip bones.

STARTING POINT

Start at the bottom of the gluteal cheek region, above the top of the back of the thigh, where the leg meets the gluteal region.

LINE OF MOVEMENT

Move up and over the buttock, toward the top of the outer hip; this may resemble the arc of a rainbow. While every buttock size is different, average three lines of movement here.

END POINT

End at the top of the outer thigh, at the side of the hip bone.

TREATMENT PROCESS

➤ Attach the cup at the starting point(s) and follow each line of movement using moving cups and/or lift-and-release to the end point. Move the cup up at a slight angle, toward the outside of the hip. Detach the cup and return to the starting point.

➤ Repeat each line of movement three to five times; in all, it takes about nine to fifteen passes to cover the entire section.

➤ Once this section is complete, continue to the next part of *Step 3, The Back of the Thighs.*

If choosing to add in the Cellulite Focus Option, proceed with that option before continuing to the next part of *Step 3.*

LOCATION NOTE

Having a difficult time locating the starting and end points?

The **starting point** is where the gluteal region begins; there is often a bubble-like bump here.

The **end point** is the end of the end point for *Step 1: The Middle and Lower Back*; it is typically directly below where you rest your hands on your hips when standing.

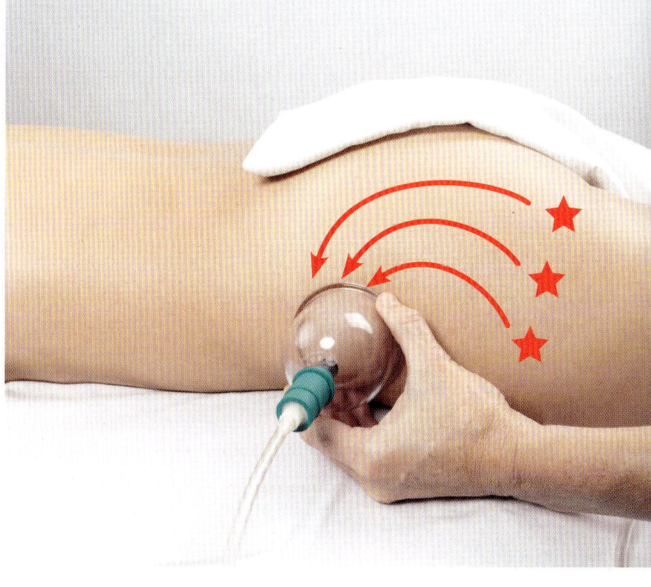

The Gluteal Region

CELLULITE FOCUS OPTION

No matter the shape and size, the buttocks are the most common area for cellulite to appear and thus a popular target for cellulite reduction. As you work around this region, be sure to keep draping (sheets or body-covering material) in place and movements comfortable, as this is a common area for overworking. While you work along the back of the gluteal region, you can add some stimulating circular movements.

After finishing the *Gluteal Region* treatment process above, use faster, vigorous movements to focus on cellulite.

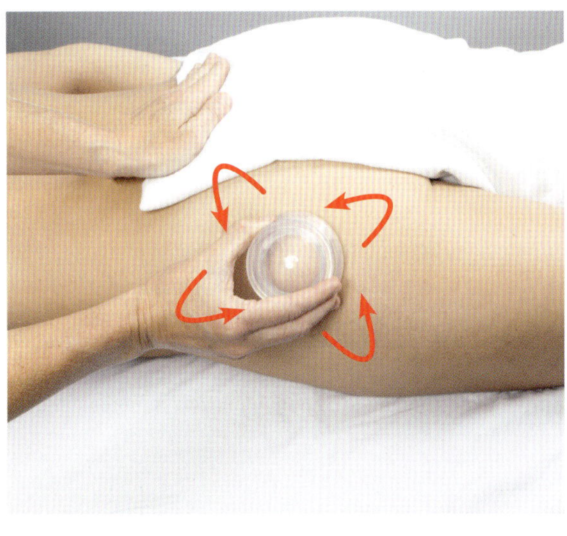

Stubborn cellulite dimples? Apply additional focused cellulite cupping as needed. Refer to page 182 for more details on these advanced methods of application.

TREATMENT PROCESS

➤ With the same lighter suction pressure, move the cup in circular movements around the buttocks at a faster yet comfortable pace.

Note: *Do not move the cup side to side while focusing on the gluteal region. While it does not go against the general flow of lymph, side-to-side here can feel odd to many people, since that direction would repetitively separate the crack line between left and right buttocks.*

➤ Repeat this fast-paced, circular movements ten to fifteen times, traveling around the entire gluteal region (see photo). Do some large circles as well as some smaller circles; these smaller circles may resemble a sketch of a daisy flower.

Suggestion: *Use one hand to anchor the gluteal region, either near the sacrum or the thigh, and the other hand to manipulate the cup. While this is not required, the recipient's buttocks may sway and move around if not held in place.*

➤ Once finished, repeat a few passes with the original, slower-paced draining lines of movement from starting point to end point.
➤ Then continue to the next part of *Step 3, The Back of the Thighs.*

The Back of the Thighs

For proper drainage flow, we divide the back of the thigh in half lengthwise. The outer half extends to the outside of the hip (the same end point as in the *Gluteal Region*) and the inner half goes to the inside end point. Both end points are considered drop-off locations when the client is lying prone, or face-down. When the client has turned over and is supine, the "dropped" material will be "picked up" and moved to the final collection areas on the front side of the body.

Begin addressing the back of the thigh just above the beginning of the back of the knee endangerment site called the popliteal fossa. (See *Chapter 4: Safe Cupping Practices*, page 71, for more detailed information.) Begin with the outer half of the thigh, then move to the inner half.

LOCATION

This area covers the back of the thigh, from above the popliteal fossa behind the knee to the buttocks.

STARTING POINT

Start just above the popliteal fossa, within the hamstring muscles. To locate the endangerment site, center one hand over the soft space in the back of the knee—this is the popliteal fossa—and begin above this space.

LINE OF MOVEMENT

Move from above the popliteal fossa, upward toward the outer and inner leg end points.

END POINT

For the outer thigh, end at the outer hip just below the hip bones; this is the same end point as the gluteal region.

For the inner thigh, end just medial to (inside) the ischial tuberosity, the lower part of the pelvis also known as the "sits bone."

SAFETY POINT

Remember: No cups should be applied directly over varicose veins. Skip over them entirely or avoid any region with excessive vascular damage. This safety rule applies to all leg applications.

The ischial tuberosities are the bony landmarks at the bottom of the ilium bones we sit on (with ideal posture).

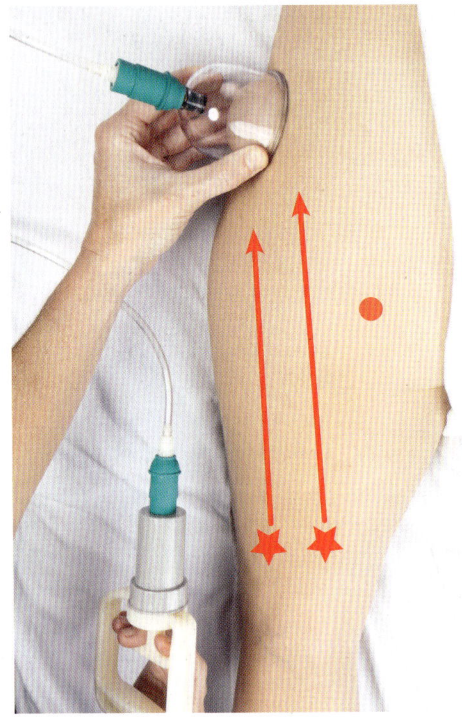

TREATMENT PROCESS

➤ Attach the cup at the starting point and follow each line of movement using moving cups and/or lift-and-release to the end points. Detach the cup and return to the starting point.

➤ *For the outer thigh* (top photo), move the cup up at a slight angle toward the outside of the hip; for a wider thigh there may be two or three lines of movement.

➤ Repeat each line of movement three to five times; while every thigh is different, there may be several passes over this lateral thigh area.

➤ Once the outer half is completed, repeat this method of application along the inner thigh.

➤ *For the inner thigh* (bottom photo), move the cup upward toward the end point.

➤ Repeat each line of movement three to five times; while every thigh is different, there may be several passes over this inner thigh area.

➤ Once the inner thigh is completed, continue to the next part of *Step 3, Stimulating the Popliteal Lymph Nodes.*

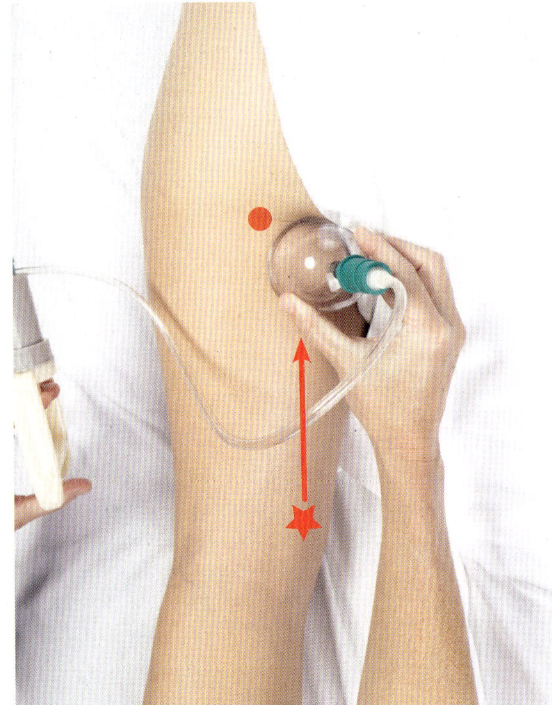

If choosing to add in the Cellulite Focus Option, proceed with that option before continuing to the next part of *Step 3.*

ABOUT PERSONAL SPACE

For the inner thigh, the end point can seem close to a person's personal, private areas. The drop-off location is near the ischial tuberosity (identified by the red dot in these photos), but still within the hamstrings at the top of the thigh. Do your best to make it not seem personally invasive. Be sure that neither your fingers nor the cup enter the person's private areas when reaching this end point. The femoral triangle (groin area) will address the fluid appropriately when brought into this region. (See *Chapter 4: Safe Cupping Practices*, page 70, for more information.)

The Back of the Thighs

CELLULITE FOCUS OPTION

The back of the thigh is often a focus area for cellulite and it can be vigorously cupped to focus on any unsightly dimples located here. This is a good location to add some side-to-side and circular movements.

After finishing the *Back of the Thighs* treatment process above, use faster, vigorous movements to focus on this region.

TREATMENT PROCESS

➤ With the same lighter suction pressure, move the cup side-to-side and/or in small, circular movements at a faster yet comfortable pace.

Note: *Do not go up and down the leg (from buttocks to knee), as that can be more sensitive than side-to-side or smaller circular movements. Up and down the leg inevitably goes against the general flow of lymph (if you move toward the knee), which can feel odd to many people.*

➤ Repeat this fast-paced, movement of choice for ten to twenty passes across the entire back of the thigh. Be sure to avoid the popliteal fossa as you work vigorously.

Suggestion: *Use one hand to anchor the leg around the knee area and the other hand to manipulate the cup. While this is not required, the recipient's leg may sway and move around if not held in place.*

➤ Once finished, repeat a few passes with the original, slower-paced draining lines of movement from starting point to end point.
➤ Then continue to the third part of *Step 3, Stimulating the Popliteal Lymph Nodes.*

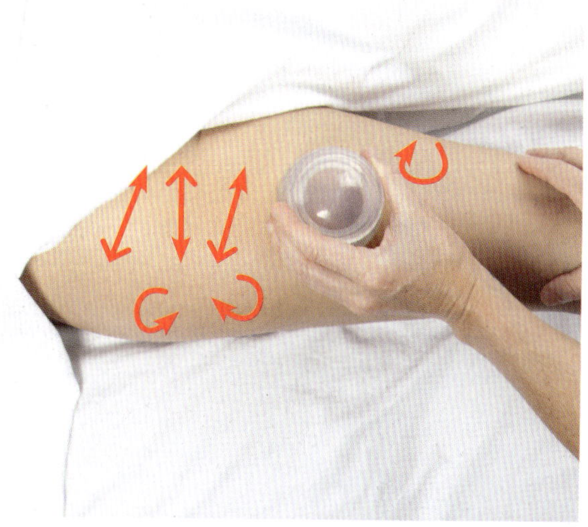

Stubborn cellulite dimples? Apply additional focused cellulite cupping as needed. Refer to page 182 for more details on these advanced methods of application.

Stimulating the Popliteal Lymph Nodes

Before moving on from the back of the leg, apply the lift-and-release technique with very light suction in the popliteal region, the soft space behind the kneecap.

LOCATION

The small area being treated is directly in the soft tissue space behind the kneecap. The starting and end points are the same.

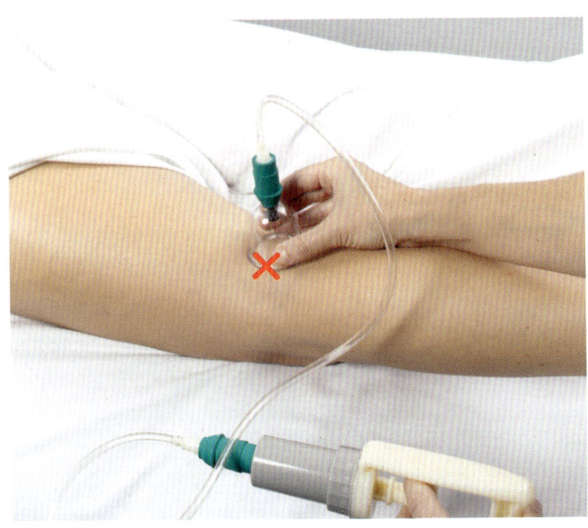

TREATMENT PROCESS

➤ Lightly apply the lift-and-release technique three to five times in the same exact location. Think of this as a gentle, therapeutic plunger.

Note: *Because this is an endangerment site, the suction should barely lift the skin.*

Once you have completed treating the left leg, treat the right leg, starting with *The Gluteal Region*, then *The Back of the Thighs* and finally, *Stimulating Popliteal Lymph Nodes*.

If adding in the *Back of the Lower Leg Option* (see page 212), do this additional step on the left before proceeding to the right leg.

After completing *Step 3* for both legs, continue to *Step 4: The Abdominal Region*.

Stimulating the Popliteal Lymph Nodes

CUP-FREE OPTION

If the cups will not work for whatever reason in this region (varicose veins, etc.) or if you prefer not to use a cup in this area, follow the Cup-Free Option, which mimics a manual lymph drainage treatment technique.

TREATMENT PROCESS

Using the same location as instructed with a cup, use your relaxed but flattened fingers to create small inward-pumping circles into the popliteal fossa.

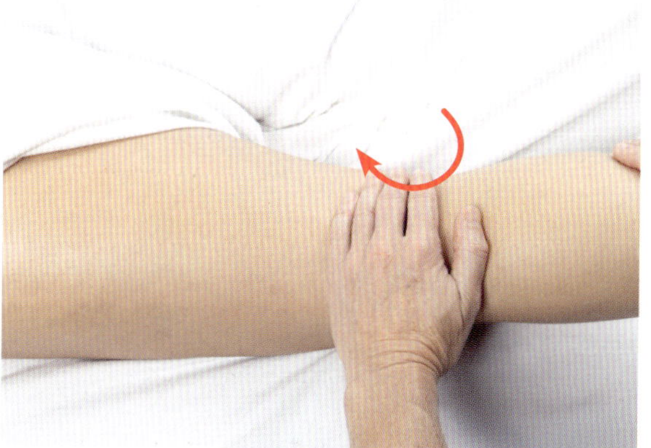

➤ Rest relaxed but flattened fingers over the popliteal fossa, and gently press softly bent fingers into the soft tissue, directing the circle up toward the hips, and out again, making a small, gentle circle into the body, upward and out again.

Note: *These circles are not meant to dig into the back of the knee. Rather, they should gently press into the skin to stimulate the regional lymph nodes located just under the skin's surface.*

➤ Repeat these gentle, skin-pressing circles three to five times in the exact same location.

Once you have completed treating the left leg, treat the right leg, starting with *The Gluteal Region*, then *The Back of the Thighs* and finally, *Stimulating Popliteal Lymph Nodes*.

After completing *Step 3* for both legs, continue to *Step 4: The Abdominal Region*.

Back of the Lower Leg Option

This optional application is not required when doing a basic full-body treatment. In lymph drainage, addressing a more proximal region (the thighs and popliteal lymph nodes) will indirectly benefit the more distal region (the lower leg).

However, it may be useful to treat the lower leg if it is an area of concern, for example, if the client experiences fluid retention or tension in the muscles located here.

Note: *Smaller cups are required to treat this area.*

LOCATION
This area focuses on the back of the lower leg below the popliteal fossa and above the ankle, commonly called the calf.

STARTING POINT
Start above the Achilles tendon, wherever a relatively larger cup can comfortably fit on the calf muscle area, usually in the thickest part of the lower leg.

LINE OF MOVEMENT
Move upward, toward the popliteal fossa. While every lower leg is different, the average calf will accommodate two lines of movement.

END POINT
End just below the popliteal fossa, within the muscles of the lower leg; be sure to not enter this endangerment site as you work through this region.

TREATMENT PROCESS

➤ Attach the cup at the starting point and follow the line of movement using moving cups and/or lift-and-release to the end point. Detach the cup, then return to the starting point.

➤ Repeat this line of movement three to five times; in all, there will be six to ten passes here.

➤ When the entire left leg has been treated, repeat the sequence of *Step 3* on the right leg.

Once you have completed *Step 3: The Back of the Lower Body* on both legs, instruct the person to turn over, face-up, for work in the supine position. Then continue to *Step 4: The Abdominal Region.*

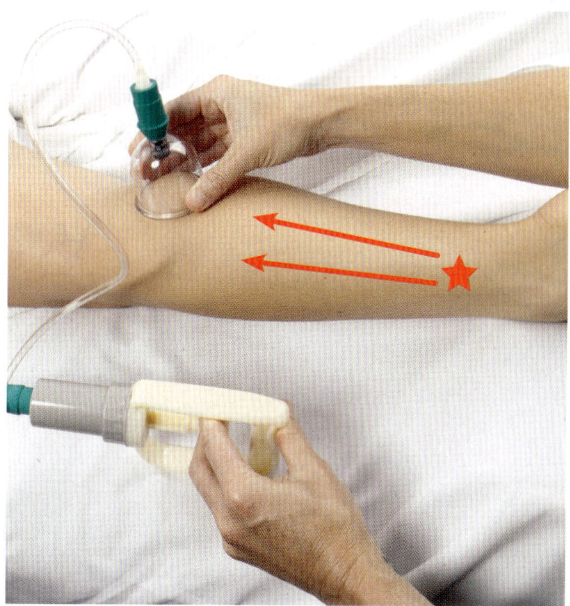

The Abdominal Region

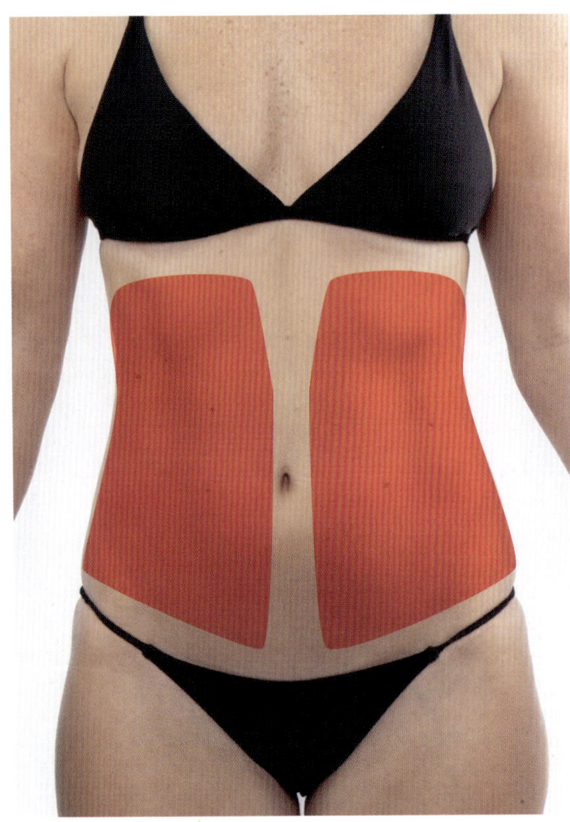

The abdomen is the most central part of the body—our core. There is a concentration of lymphatic activity in this region. Because of that, working in this region is a vital part of a full-body lymphatic drainage treatment. Also, as much tension and congestion often exist within the abdomen, it is a very common site for body contouring and cellulite treatments.

Note: *For all of Step 4 and the remaining steps, the person being treated is in the supine, face-up position.*

WHY CUP THE ABDOMEN?

Cupping through the abdomen is incredibly therapeutic on many levels, providing relief from lymphatic congestion to muscle tension and digestive issues. Using the cups to follow lymph pathways promotes softness and definition in this often-tense region, all without the positive pressure of pressing into the abdomen.

And although this is a common location for cellulite, any focused cupping here is done with more repetitive passes over the region rather than vigorous movements. Vigorous movement is best avoided in this area.

For greatest benefit, we divide this region into two parts: *Stimulating the Upper Inguinal Lymph Nodes* and *Contouring the Abdomen.* We end this step with a quick manual treatment, *Finishing the Abdomen.*

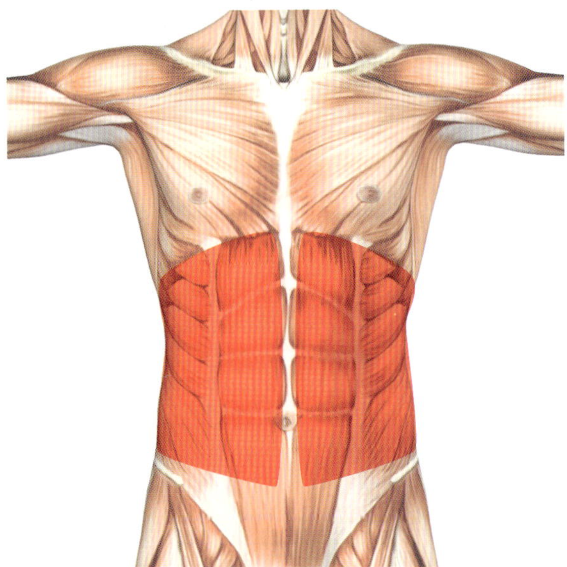

Stimulating the Upper Inguinal Lymph Nodes in the supine position is necessary to collect all the drained lymph material that was dropped off along the sides of the body in *Step 1* and to prepare the abdomen for the rest of the treatment. These lymph nodes are superficial, yet connect to deeper nodes and drainage vessels within the abdominal region. Beginning the abdominal region with this quick lift-and-release stimulates the upper inguinal lymph nodes to "unclog the drain" in the lower abdomen; after this, all lines of movement end in the same location to deposit the lymph "garbage."

Contouring the Abdomen gently yet effectively smooths the abdominal space. With every movement, tissues will soften and relax, allowing fascial tension to ease, adipose to contour without discomfort and lymph to move more freely through the area. The starting points here will pick up the lymph materials that were dropped off at the sides when treating the posterior midsection (the *Middle and Lower Back*), and will continue the drainage to its final collection area in the lower abdomen, while addressing the entire abdomen, too. Cupping through here is often sensitive and may feel "sticky" at first, so be sure to use lift-and-release and the combination Morse Code of Cups as needed to make every line of movement smooth and comfortable. Remember that moving cups work best with light suction, and since there are many vital visceral organs here, be sure not to force any restrictions you encounter as you work along each line of movement. There is also a Cellulite Focus Option for this part of *Step 4*.

Finishing the Abdomen, the final part of this step, is a gentle manual treatment that encourages colon circulation.

SAFETY FIRST

The abdomen is one of the most sensitive areas of the body and there are many potential reasons why cupping or general bodywork should be avoided. Some contraindications to cupping include separation of the abdominal muscles (diastasis recti), hernias and unknown abdominal pains.

Also, the abdomen contains many visceral organs and specialized adipose tissue that can easily become inflamed if overworked. For these reasons, be sure to follow instructions carefully to ensure best and safe results.

TRUE MLD THERAPY VERSUS CUPPING FOR BODY CONTOURING

In the abdomen, there are two drainage regions for manual lymph drainage (MLD) therapies. The transverse watershed divides the torso into *inguinal regions* (which drain the midsection and lower half of the torso) and the *axillary regions* (which drain the top half of the torso).

In the treatment described here, some lines of movement may cross this watershed division. For the generally well person, this is not an issue and is totally safe when done in the order described in this book (starting at the hip bones and progressing upward).

This method of treatment is comparable to how MLD can enable *anastomoses*, which is a lymphatic component that allows for alternate routes of lymph drainage safely.

In this treatment process we focus on contouring in the abdomen in a basic manner. MLD therapists are welcome to adjust treatment instructions to follow their advanced training. Both methods of application are safe, effective and will yield great results.

Stimulating the Upper Inguinal Lymph Nodes

Begin treating the abdomen by stimulating the upper inguinal lymph nodes to receive lymph from the midsection.

LOCATION

This area is just above the anterior superior iliac spine hip points within the abdominal muscle, on the left and right sides of the abdomen. Generally, this is in the lower two muscle segments of the rectus abdomimus muscles, the bottom two portions of the "six pack." Everything happens in the same location, so there is no separate starting point or end point.

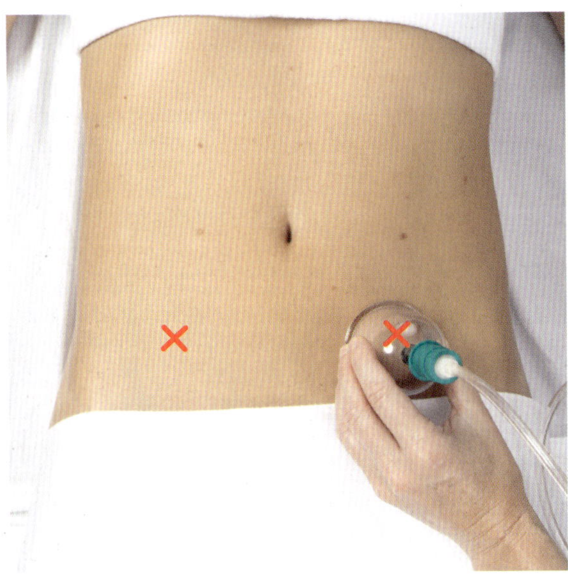

TREATMENT PROCESS

➤ Lightly apply the lift-and-release technique three to five times in the exact same location. Think of this as a gentle, therapeutic plunger.

➤ Repeat this sequence on the right side of the body, then continue to the next part of *Step 3, Contouring the Abdomen.*

Because this location is not within an endangerment site, there is no Cup-Free Option.

Contouring the Abdomen

Begin addressing the abdomen in the lower region, just above the anterior superior iliac spine. As you progress, the entire abdominal region will be treated, ending below the breast tissue and over the lower rib cage.

LOCATION

This area is within the midsection of the body, from hip bones to the lower rib cage; be sure to stay below the breast tissue.

STARTING POINT

Start along the side of the body, just above the hip bones. This is the end point from the start of *Step 1*, where you dropped off lymph.

LINE OF MOVEMENT

Move from the side of the body, into the lower abdomen end point(s). Be sure to keep the body divided in half lengthwise; move from left side to left end point, right side to right end point.

END POINT

End at the upper inguinal lymph nodes; the same location that is stimulated at the beginning of this step.

TREATMENT PROCESS

➤ Attach the cup lightly at the starting point and follow the line of movement using moving cups and/or lift-and-release to the end point. Detach the cup and return to the starting point.

➤ Repeat this line of movement three to five times.

➤ Once cup-width at a time, progress up the midsection, continuing to the same end point in the lower abdomen every time.

➤ End just below the breast tissue, working over the lower rib cage.

➤ Once you have completed this side, repeat the *Contouring the Abdomen* process on the right side of the abdomen.

PROPER LINE OF MOVEMENT

Be sure to keep the body divided in half lengthwise; move from the left side of the abdomen in toward the left lower drop-off location, and from the right side of the abdomen toward the right lower drop-off location.

If choosing to add in the Cellulite Focus Option, proceed with that option before continuing to the next part of Step 5.

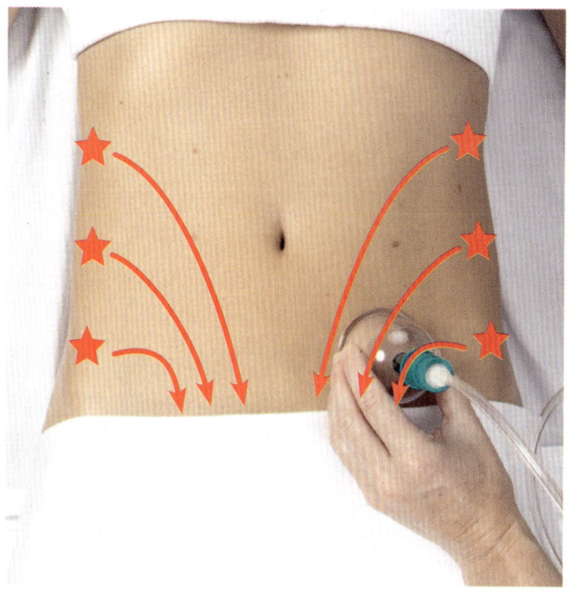

Contouring the Abdomen

CELLULITE FOCUS OPTION

Unlike other parts of the body where cellulite focus is done with different methods of application, in the abdomen the only way to focus is by repeating the same lines of movement multiple times. There should be no vigorous movements in any direction, and no more focused applications as suggested elsewhere. Considering the delicate anatomy in the abdominal region, simply repeating the treatment process a few additional times will safely and effectively add to the contouring of the abdomen.

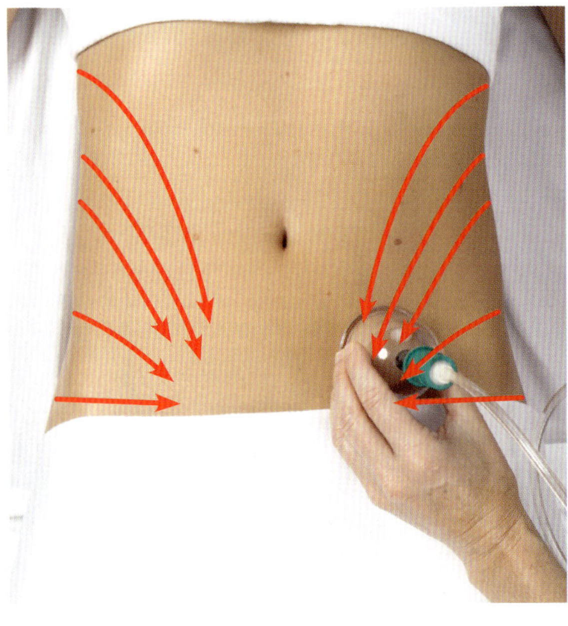

TREATMENT PROCESS

➤ To focus on cellulite in the abdomen, simply follow the same lines of movement described for the Contouring the Abdomen treatment process several more times.

➤ You may repeat these draining lines of movement ten or twenty times in total, including the original three to five passes. With every pass, you will see contour becoming more defined.

Note: *Be sure not to overwork this area, as the abdomen contains subcutaneous adipose tissue that can easily become irritated if overworked. Some people have specialized adipose tissue (panniculus) in the lower abdominal area, which can easily become inflamed if overworked, causing it to thicken more than it already is. Deeper into the abdomen is visceral fat, which wraps and protects the organs contained within this region.*

INDICATIONS OF ENOUGH CUPPING

The skin will most likely pinken while you cup the abdomen, indicating significantly increased blood flow. However, if it becomes red or extremely warm to touch, that is enough cupping for the session. Also, people may report becoming sensitive or experiencing discomfort if the area is overworked, as this is a response to overstimulation of the nerve endings in the area.

Finishing the Abdomen

After you have finished treating both sides of the abdomen, put down the cup and use your hands to gently follow the length of the entire colon two or three times.

Why? Part of this abdominal treatment travels against the flow of the colon (on the client's right side), so doing this quick cup-free application will ensure happy, healthy colon circulation, and is a nice way to finish cupping through the abdomen.

This treatment is done with light and lymphatic intentions; there is no need to add much pressure into the abdomen.

LOCATION

The colon starts in the lower right abdomen, travels up toward the right side of the rib cage (ascending colon), across the abdomen toward the left side of the rib cage (transverse colon), down toward the left hip bones (descending colon) and then bends back toward the midline, finishing about one hand-width below the belly button (sigmoid colon and rectum).

TREATMENT PROCESS

➤ Starting in their left midsection (addressing the descending colon), began applying circular movements in a clockwise direction within the entire abdominal section. This is the exact same method of abdominal massage that began the entire treatment in *The Preliminary Steps*.

➤ Repeat these circular movements five to ten times.

➤ Once the abdominal region is completed, continue to *Step 5: The Front of the Legs*.

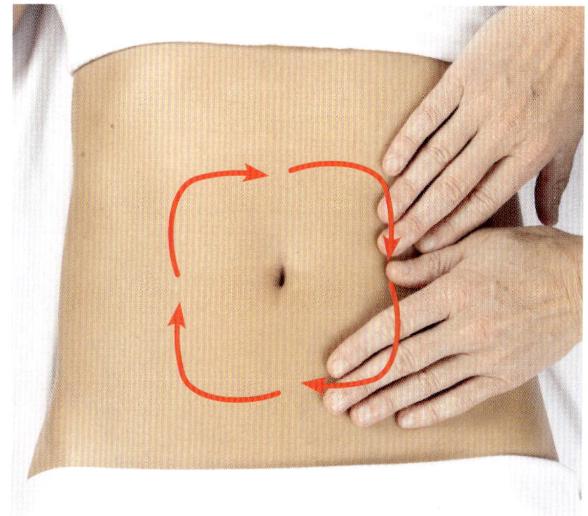

The Front of the Legs

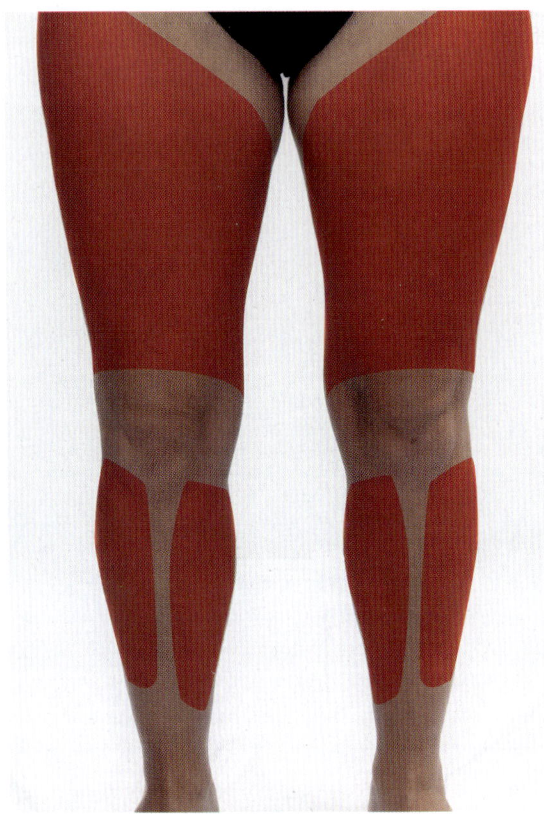

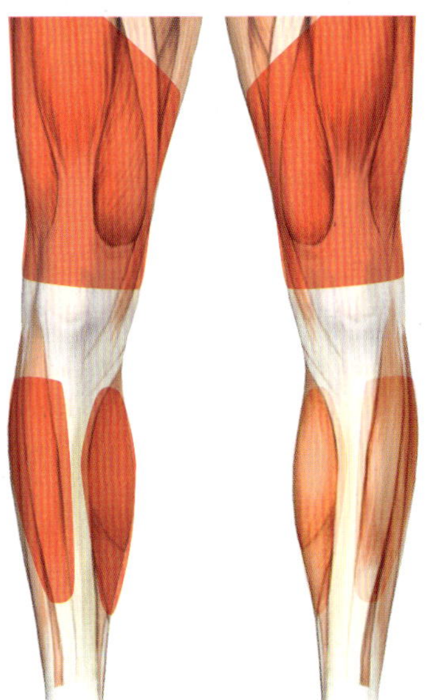

Whether there is lymphatic congestion due to a sedentary lifestyle, muscle tension, an injury contributing to the restrictions or simply an area in need of some smoothing, the front of the leg benefits greatly from lymphatic drainage and contouring.

WHY CUP THE FRONT OF THE LEGS?

Cupping the front of the legs helps move lymph through this often compressed region and relax muscle tension in the front of the thighs.

For greatest benefit, we divide this region into two parts: *Stimulating the Lower Inguinal Lymph Nodes* and *The Front of the Thighs*. There is also a *Front of the Lower Leg Option* for this step.

Stimulating the Lower Inguinal Lymph Nodes is necessary to collect all the drained lymph material that is moved along the leg, in both prone and supine positions. These lower inguinal lymph nodes are located within the femoral triangle and personal groin spaces. Stimulating this region is another "unclogging the drain" step that helps drainage from the lower body move upward. There is also a Cup-Free Option for this part of *Step 5*.

The Front of the Thighs covers all the area above the knees on the front side of the leg, including inner and outer thigh areas. Working through this area will collect the materials that were dropped off at *Step 3* end points, "scooping" the fluids from the outer hip and thigh areas inward toward the groin. Cupping here is also a great way to work through the long quadricep and adductor muscles of the upper leg, ironing out any lumps and bumps that exist here. There is also a Cellulite Focus Option for this part of *Step 5*.

Stimulating the Lower Inguinal Lymph Nodes

Begin treating the front of the leg by addressing the upper inner thigh; this stimulates the lower inguinal lymph nodes to receive lymph from the leg.

Note: *The cup does not need to be all the way up into the person's private groin area. Cupping within the femoral triangle will suffice. Considering the effect cups have over general areas, lymph can be stimulated from a comfortable distance, about a hand-width distance from the groin area.*

LOCATION

The area to be treated is at the top of the thigh, about one hand-width from the groin, and along the inner part of the upper thigh. This is within the femoral triangle endangerment site. Since everything occurs in the same location, there is no separate starting point or end point.

TREATMENT PROCESS

➤ Lightly apply the lift-and-release technique three to five times in the exact same location. Think of this as a gentle, therapeutic plunger.

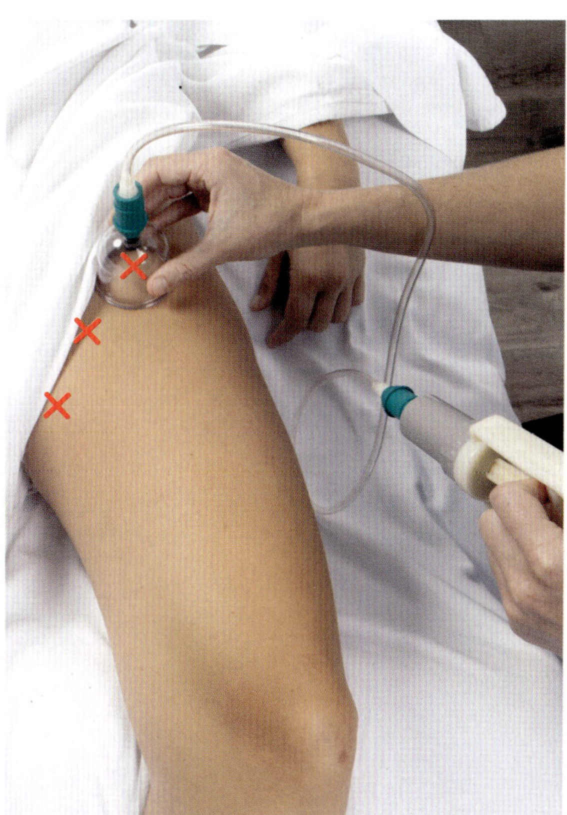

Stimulating the Lower Inguinal Lymph Nodes

CUP-FREE OPTION

If the cups will not work for whatever reason in this region (too close for personal comfort, etc.) or if you prefer not to use a cup in this area, follow the Cup-Free Option, which mimics a manual lymph drainage treatment technique.

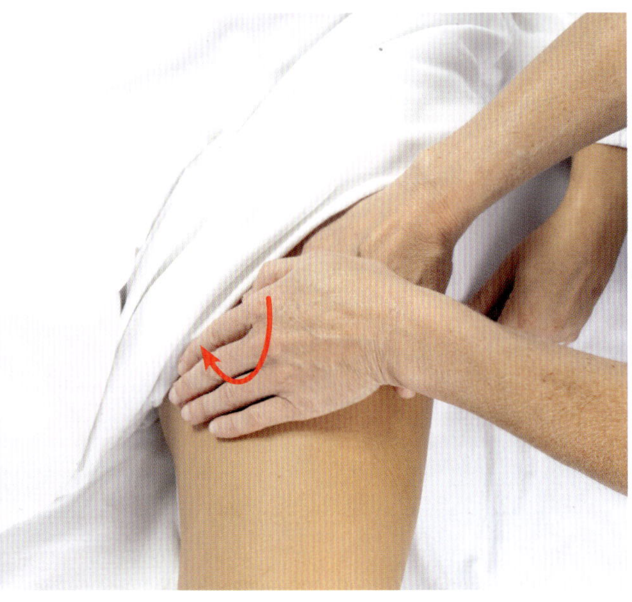

TREATMENT PROCESS

Using the same location as instructed with a cup, use your relaxed but flattened fingers and the palm of your hand to create small inward and upward pumping circles, in the direction of the groin.

➤ Rest relaxed but flattened fingers and palms at the femoral triangle region; you can stack hands or simply use one hand to do this in such a personal, private space.
➤ Gently press flattened fingers and palm into the skin and upward toward the groin area, making a small, gentle circle into the body and out again.

Note: *These circles are not meant to dig into the groin. Rather, they should gently press into the skin to stimulate the regional lymph nodes located just under the skin's surface.*

➤ Repeat these gentle, skin-pressing circles three to five times in the exact same location.
➤ Once this section is completed, proceed to the next part of *Step 5: The Front of the Thighs.*

The Front of the Thighs

Begin addressing the front of the thigh just above the knee. Each line of movement will address the entire front of upper leg region, so, depending on the size of the thigh, there may be three, four, five or more lines of movement per thigh.

As our example, we have assumed four lines of movement to cover the entire front of the upper leg. That is why there are four starting points and four lines of movement shown.

LOCATION

This area is from the top of the knee to the hip bones, and from the outermost part of the thigh to the inner thigh.

STARTING POINT

1. *The outer hip* starts at the top outside of the hip, below the hip bones but at the top of the thigh. This scoops fluids forward from the drop-off location in *Step 3*, the back of the outer thigh.
2. *The outer thigh* will start above the outer part of the knee. This may be very sticky or sensitive, as it travels over the iliotibial band, commonly known as the IT band.
3. *The midline of the thigh* will start directly above the knee.
4. *The inner thigh* will start directly above the inner part of the knee.

LINE OF MOVEMENT

1. Move across the upper thigh, toward the groin.
2. Move along the outer line of the thigh, up toward the hip and the groin; you will notice a slight angle as you approach the top of the thigh.
3. Move along the top of the thigh, toward the groin.
4. Move along the inner thigh, toward the groin.

END POINT

Each line of movement ends at the femoral triangle area, where you began this step, *Stimulating the Lower Inguinal Lymph Nodes*.

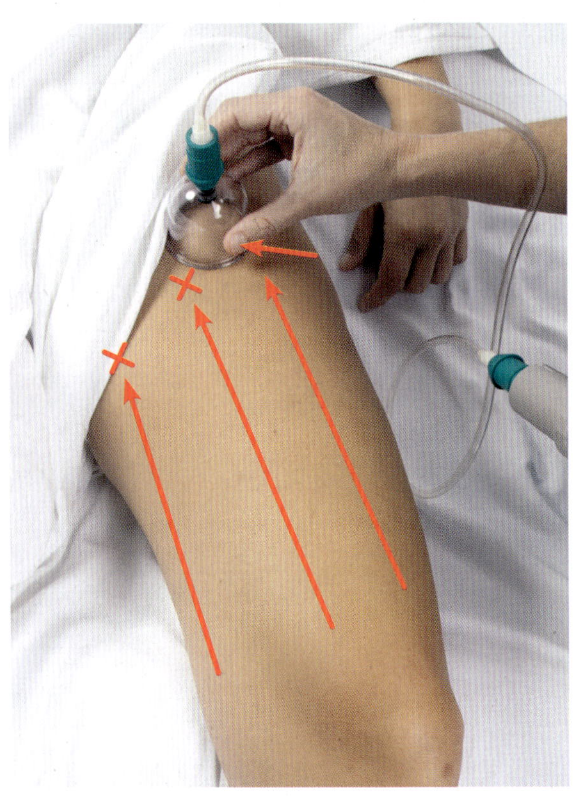

TREATMENT PROCESS

➤ Attach the cup at each starting point and follow each line of movement using moving cups and/or lift-and-release to the end point. Detach the cup and return to the starting point.

➤ Repeat each line of movement three to five times; in all, there will be at least twelve to twenty lines of movement.

Note: *Use the lift-and-release technique to move over any sensitive areas comfortably if necessary.*

If choosing to add in the Cellulite Focus Option, proceed with that option before continuing on to *Step 6*.

The Front of the Thighs

CELLULITE FOCUS OPTION

This location is often a focus area for cellulite and can be vigorously cupped to focus on any unsightly dimples located here. Treating the entire front of the thigh will address the front of the thighs and the inner thighs, as well as the outer thighs, commonly called "saddlebags." While you work over the front of the thigh, this is a good location to add some side-to-side and circular movements.

After finishing the treatment process above, use faster, vigorous movements to focus on this region.

TREATMENT PROCESS

➤ With the same lighter suction pressure, move the cup side to side and/or in small, circular movements at a faster yet comfortable pace.

Note: *Do not go up and down the leg (from the top of the thigh to the knee), as that can be more sensitive than side-to-side or smaller circular movements. Up and down the leg inevitably goes against the general flow of lymph (if you move toward the knee), which can feel odd to many people.*

➤ Repeat these fast-paced vigorous movements of choice for ten to twenty passes across the entire front of the thigh. Be sure to work mindfully around the groin area as you work.

Suggestion: *Use one hand to anchor the leg around the knee area and the other hand to manipulate the cup. While this is not required, the recipient's leg may sway and move around if not held in place.*

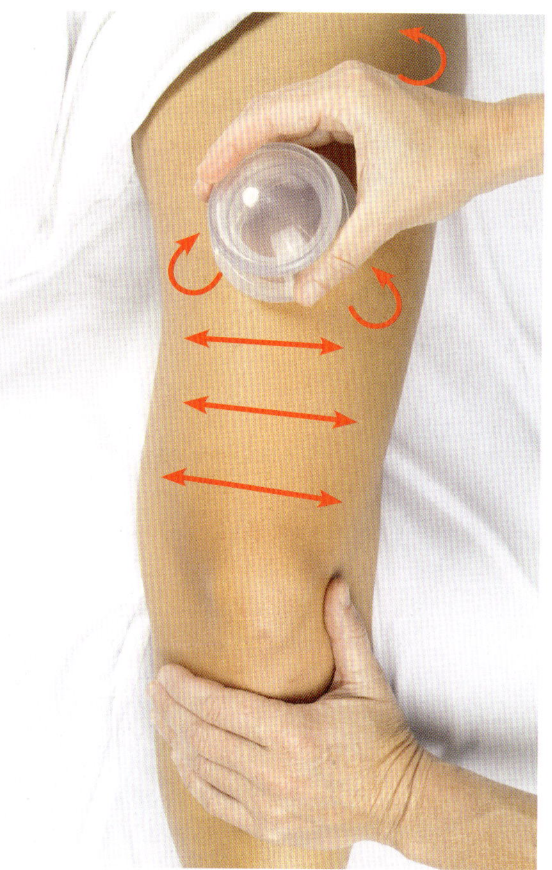

Stubborn cellulite dimples? Apply additional focused cellulite cupping as needed. Refer to page 182 for more details on these advanced methods of application.

Inner thigh suggestion: *To focus here, consider rotating the recipient's leg open to the side, maybe using a pillow to offer additional support, and be sure the draping remains in place for personal comfort.*

➤ Once finished, repeat a few passes with the original, slower-paced draining lines of movement from starting point to end point.

➤ Then continue to *Step 6: The Front of the Arms and Chest.*

If adding in the *Front of the Lower Leg Option* (see page 227), do this additional step before proceeding to the other leg. After completing *Step 5* for both legs, continue to *Step 6: The Front of the Arms and Chest.*

Front of the Lower Leg Option

This optional application is not required for a basic full-body treatment. In lymph drainage, addressing a more proximal region (the front of the thighs) will indirectly benefit the more distal region (the lower leg). However, it may be useful to treat the lower leg if it is an area of concern, for example, if your client experiences fluid retention or tension in the muscles located here.

Note: *Smaller cups are required to treat this area.*

LOCATION
The area of treatment is the front of lower leg, divided in half lengthwise by the tibia, or shinbone, for two lines of movement.

STARTING POINT
Start above the ankle bones; first address the inner lower leg on the inside and then address the outside of the lower leg.

LINE OF MOVEMENT
Move along the length of the lower leg, up toward the knee, first along the inside and then along the outside.

END POINT
End just below the knee, on the inside and outside of the leg.

TREATMENT PROCESS
➤ Attach the cup at the starting point(s) and follow the line(s) of movement using moving cups and/or lift-and-release to the end point(s). Detach the cup and return to the starting point(s).

➤ Repeat each line of movement along the inside and outside of lower leg three to five times.

➤ When the entire left leg has been treated, repeat the sequence of *Step 5* on the right leg.

➤ Once both legs have been treated, continue to *Step 6: The Front of the Arms and Chest.*

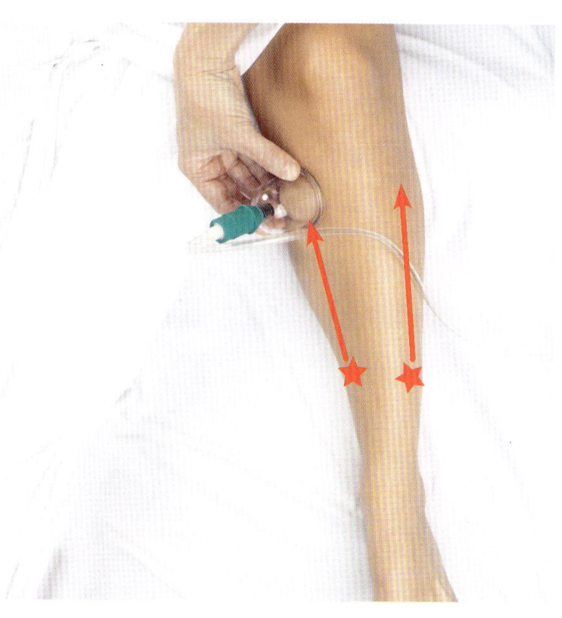

The Front of the Arms and Chest

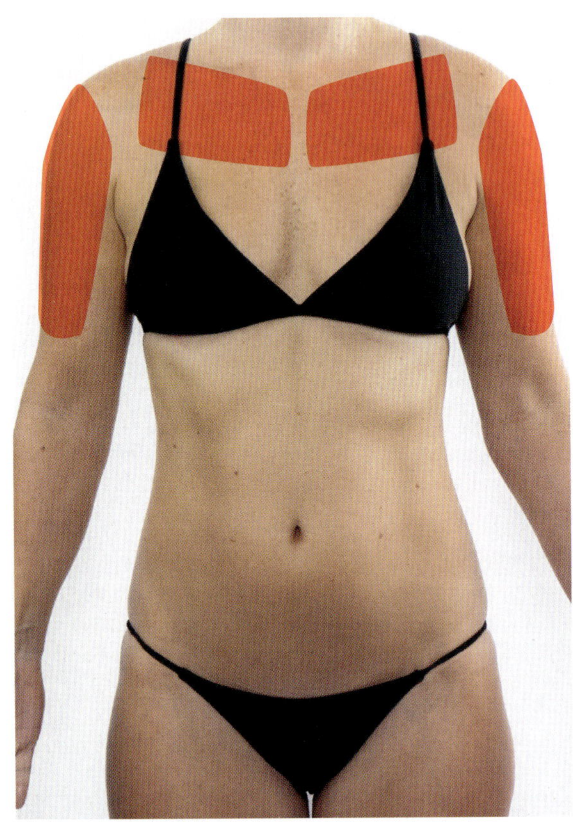

When finishing the full-body treatment, the last region we address is the upper chest and the front of the arms (if necessary). Even though the focus on cellulite is low in this region, the lymphatic activity is high. That means the best way to finish the entire treatment is to work through this upper body area.

WHY CUP THE UPPER ARMS AND CHEST?

Cupping through this area concludes the lymphatic drainage processes, and is a wonderful way to clear any lingering tension from the front of the upper body.

For greatest benefit, we divide this region into four parts: *Stimulating the Axillary Lymph Nodes*, *The Front of the Upper Arms*, *Stimulating the Thoracic Lymph Nodes* and *The Upper Chest Finishing Move*.

Stimulating the Axillary Lymph Nodes will further activate the lymphatic activity in the upper body. Yes, this area was already stimulated in *Step 2,* but it is important to revisit this area when finishing all the lymphatic drainage across the front of the body. As lymph flows, most of the chest drains out toward the axilla, too, so stimulating this region is a great way to "unclog the drain" as the final sections are drained. There is also a Cup-Free Option for this part of this step.

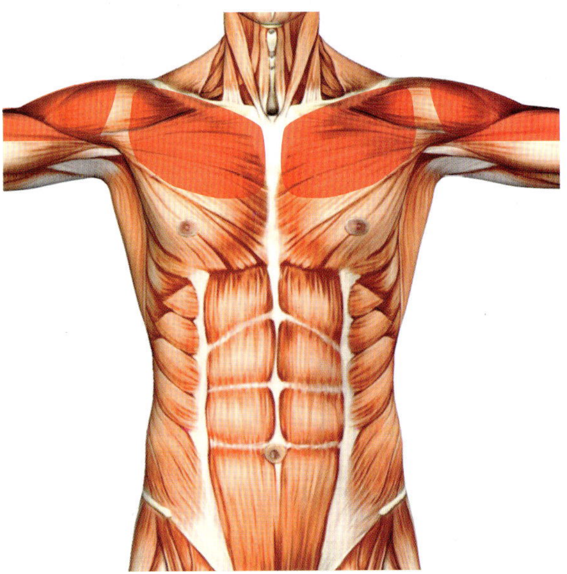

The Front of the Upper Arm is a very small area. You can consider treating it in this position, while your client is face-up. While most of the upper arm was treated during *Step 2*, if there is more area to address on the front side of the arm, this is the best way to do so. Consider this an optional part of this step if most of the upper arm was covered in *Step 2*; there is no need to go over this same area again.

Stimulating the Thoracic Lymph Nodes is a must after such a powerful, full-body treatment is complete. While some of this region was stimulated before *Step 1* began, it is the ultimate end point for all lymph drainage of the body, and therefore the best way to finish such a thorough lymphatic treatment.

The Upper Chest Finishing Move is the final step in this entire process. As the lymphatic system works, the upper chest drains out toward the axilla, and the circuit of drainage completes its cycle from there. This region also contributes to general shoulder tension, so gently using cups across the upper chest is very relaxing to the often-tense muscles located here.

Lower Arm Treatment?

Considering the focus of this book is on cellulite reduction and body contouring, the lower arm treatment is omitted from the treatment process. Don't worry that omitting this region will mean the total lymphatic drainage is not complete. Remember, treating the upper arm will directly benefit lower arm drainage—clearing a proximal area (the upper arm and axilla regions are closer to the center of the body) before a distal area (the lower arm) has a direct effect on distal lymphatic drainage activity.

SAFETY FIRST

VASCULAR CONSIDERATIONS IN THE UPPER CHEST AND ARM

Although they are not endangerment sites, the front of the shoulder and upper chest contain many blood vessels and nerves that deserve consideration as you work in this area. The many branches of arteries and veins (subclavian, brachial, axillary, cephalic, basilic) as well as the brachial plexus of nerves travel through this region; often the veins are visible just under the skin here.

Be mindful of the anatomy as you travel through this region.

Stimulating the Axillary Lymph Nodes

Begin stimulating these regional lymph nodes by working in the armpit endangerment site with very light suction pressure.

LOCATION
The area being treated is within the soft tissue space of the armpit.

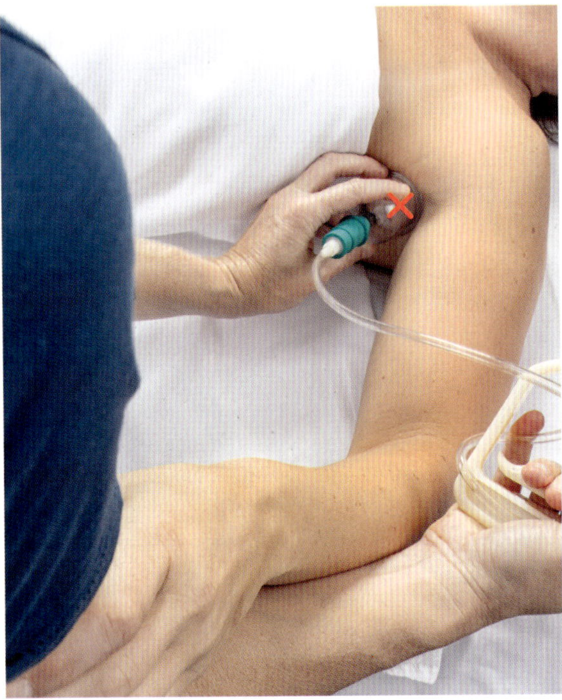

TREATMENT PROCESS
- Lightly apply the lift-and-release technique three to five times in the same exact location. Think of this as a gentle, therapeutic plunger.
- Once one axilla has been stimulated, repeat this process in the other axilla.

Note: *Because this is an endangerment site, the suction should barely lift the skin.*

Stimulating the Axillary Lymph Nodes

CUP-FREE OPTION

If the cups will not work for whatever reason in this region (excessive body hair, etc.) or if you prefer not to use a cup in this area, follow the Cup-Free Option, which mimics a manual lymph drainage treatment technique.

TREATMENT PROCESS

Using the same location as instructed with a cup, use your relaxed but flattened fingers to create small inward-pumping circles into the axilla. If standing at the head of the table, consider stimulating both axillary lymph nodes at the same time, using both hands (one hand in each axillary space). If not, follow the instructions for one axilla, then stimulate the other.

> Rest relaxed but flattened fingers at the armpit region, and gently flex the fingers into the armpit and out again, making a small, gentle circle into the body and out again.

Note: *The circles are done in toward the torso and back out again. These circles are not meant to dig into the armpit. Rather, they should gently press into the skin to stimulate the regional lymph nodes located just under the skin's surface.*

> Repeat these gentle, skin-pressing circles three to five times in each location.
> Once this section is completed, proceed to the next part of *Step 6, The Front of the Upper Arms.*

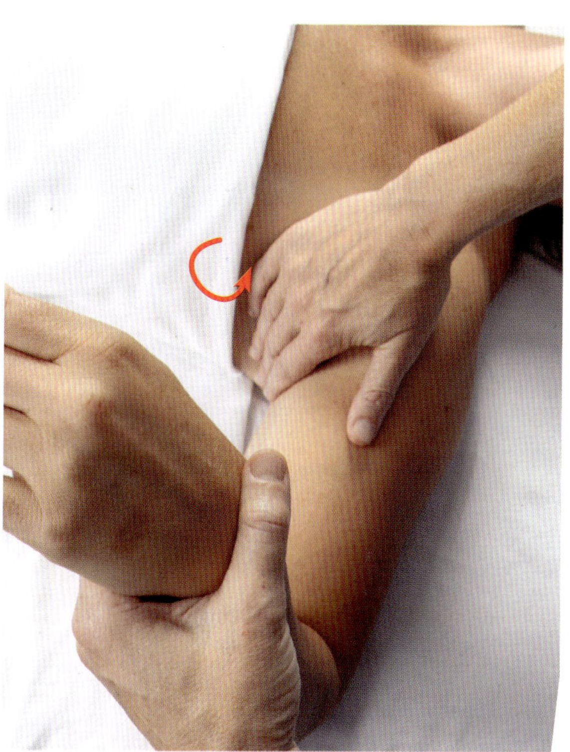

The Front of the Upper Arms

Begin addressing the upper arm just above the elbow.

LOCATION
This area includes the front side of the upper arm, whatever was not treated in *Step 2*. Typically, this is the biceps muscle.

STARTING POINT
Start just above the elbow.

LINE OF MOVEMENT
Move along the front of the upper arm, toward the armpit.

END POINT
End in front of the armpit; be sure not to move into the axilla, as it is an endangerment site.

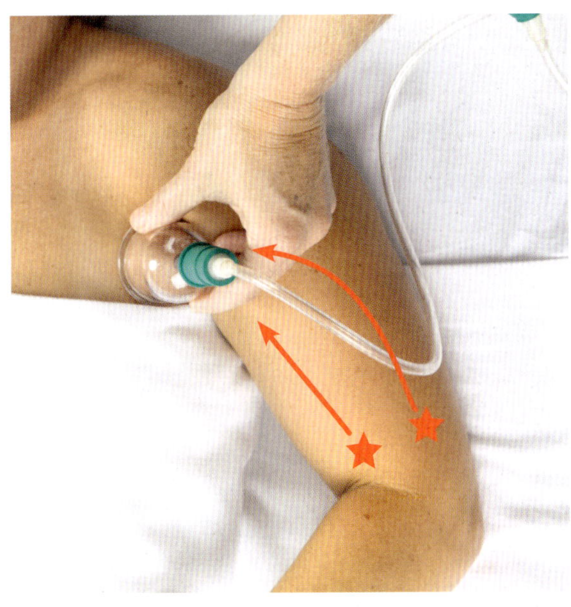

TREATMENT PROCESS
➤ Attach the cup at the starting point and follow the line of movement using moving cups and/or lift-and-release to the end point. Detach the cup and return to the starting point.

Note: *This may be a sensitive line of movement or difficult to slide because of tight muscles, so use the lift-and-release technique to move over this area comfortably if necessary.*

➤ Repeat this line of movement three to five times.

Once the left arm has been treated, repeat these first two parts of *Step 6* for the other upper arm.

Stimulating the Thoracic Lymph Nodes

Begin treating the chest by stimulating the thoracic lymph nodes. This action helps to assimilate all the lymph fluids moved during this full-body lymphatic drainage cupping treatment.

LOCATION

The area being treated is just below the sternoclavicular notch in the center of the chest, on the left and right respectively. This area is approximately the size of all flattened fingers across the upper chest, starting at the sternum in the center and over toward the axilla, but no further than the middle underside of the clavicle.

TREATMENT PROCESS

➤ Lightly apply the lift-and-release technique three to five times in the exact same location. Think of this as a gentle, therapeutic plunger.

➤ Repeat this sequence on the right side of the body, then continue to the last part of *Step 6, The Upper Chest Finishing Move.*

Considering this location is not within an endangerment site, there is no Cup-Free Option.

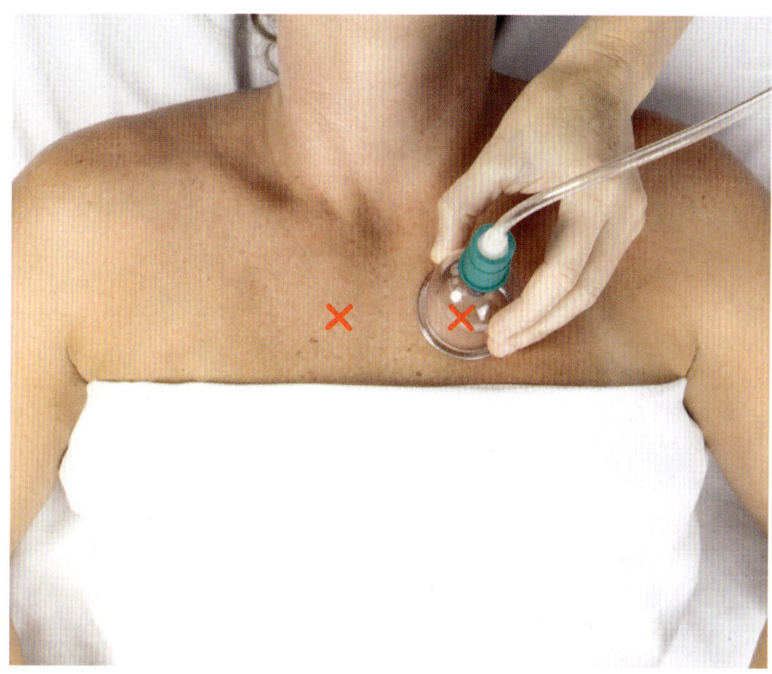

The Upper Chest Finishing Move

This finishing move addresses the upper chest just below the clavicle, or collarbones. It will help to clear the region and boost all lymphatic activity.

LOCATION
The area being treated is below the clavicle but above the breast tissue, from sternum centerline out to axilla.

STARTING POINT
Start in the midline of the chest below the sternoclavicular notch but within the pectoral muscle and just off center, left and right respectively.

LINE OF MOVEMENT
Move from the midline of the chest, across the upper chest region, toward the axilla.

END POINT
End at the outermost part of the upper chest, just before entering the axilla endangerment site.

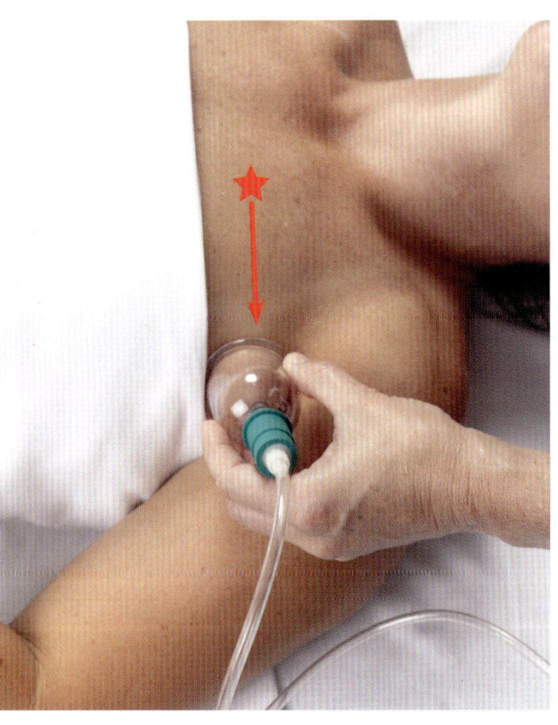

TREATMENT PROCESS
➤ Attach the cup lightly at the starting point and follow the lines of movement with moving cups and/or lift-and-release to the end point. Detach the cup and return to the starting point.
➤ Repeat this line of movement three to five times.

Note: *This region contains many prominent blood vessels close to the surface; be sure to not work too aggressively if they are very prominent.*

➤ Repeat this sequence on the right side of the upper chest.

This step completes the full-body cupping treatment.

THE BODY-CUPPING MAP

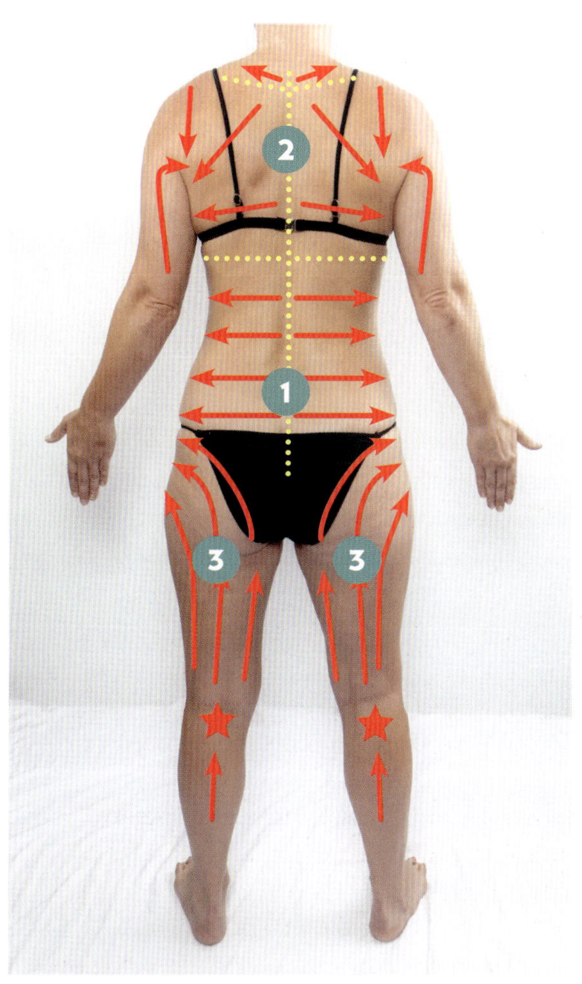
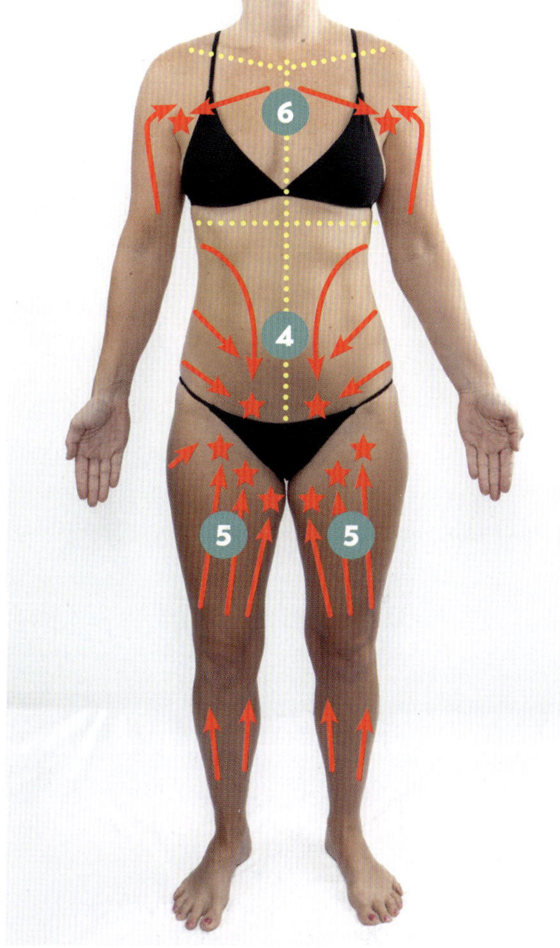

LEGEND

1 The Middle and Lower Back (page 191)

2 The Back of the Upper Body (page 194)

3 The Back of the Lower Body (page 203)

4 The Abdominal Region (page 214)

5 The Front of the Legs (page 220)

6 The Front of the Arms and Chest (page 228)

BODY CUPPING FOR SELF-CARE

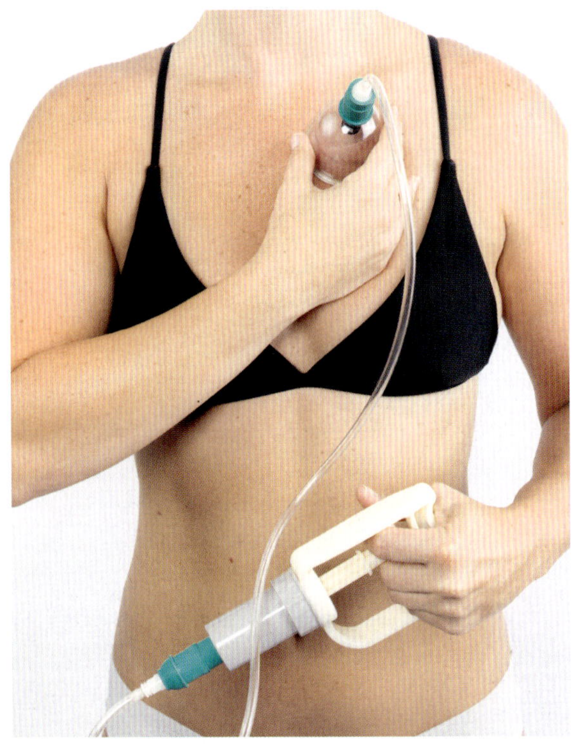

It can be challenging to treat the entire body during a self-care treatment. It is easiest to stand up during a self-care application. However, for the abdomen, you will want to lie down so the muscles can relax. Getting at every location comfortably can be tricky, but do the best you can.

At the very least, focus on the central regions of your own body—your midsection, then hips and thighs above knees, then chest and arms above elbows—for the best outcome. See *Quick-Fix Cellulite Shortcuts*, on the next page, for more information on this self-care shortcut option.

WHAT CUPS TO USE

Manual pump cups offer a great deal of mobility but require that cups be held properly. Because the hand pump handle is easy to use, this type of cupping equipment may be more comfortable for most self-care purposes.

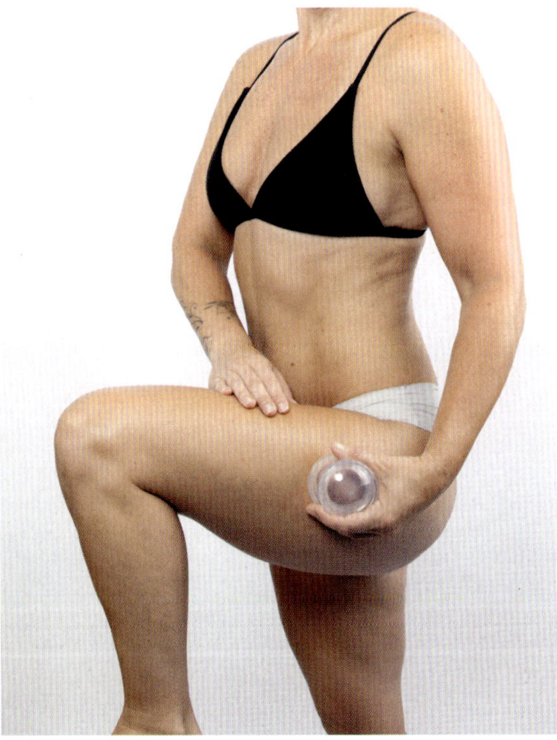

Silicone cups are easy to grip and to move because of their indentations. They require repetitive squeezing action, however, which can be difficult for some users. If for self-care, these are recommended for any cellulite focus areas.

QUICK-FIX CELLULITE SHORTCUTS

This cellulite reduction treatment is most effective when the entire body is treated, from knees to elbows—the core of the body, as well as the more cellulite-affected parts of the extremities. As a rule, doing a full-body treatment is the best way to boost overall circulation for applications that focus on cellulite reduction.

And yet, it is understood that some people just want to "cup and go" for cellulite reduction. While this is not ideal, choosing to address focus areas only is possible if you acknowledge the lymphatic system and its holistic approach to its drainage. In other words, that means if you just want to focus on the gluteals and thighs, you still have to stimulate lymph nodes within that drainage region, and make sure to follow the instructions for that body part.

QUICK-FIX TREATMENT PROCESS

➤ **To focus on midsection and abdomen**, do *Step 1* and *Step 4*. But first, be sure to *Stimulate the Upper Inguinal Lymph Nodes* before you begin, then do *Step 1* and then *Step 4*. You will stimulate the upper inguinal lymph node areas twice. (See pages 216, 192 and 218.)

➤ **To focus on the thighs and gluteal region**, do *Step 3* and *Step 5*. But first, be sure to *Stimulate the Upper and Lower Inguinal Lymph Node* areas before you begin, then do *Step 3* and then *Step 5*. You will stimulate both inguinal lymph node areas twice. (See pages 216, 221, 205 , 208 and 224.)

➤ **To focus on the arms**, do part of *Step 2* and *Step 6*. But first, be sure to *Stimulate the Axillary and Thoracic Lymph Node* areas before you begin, then do part of *Step 2* (the *Upper Arms*) and then *Step 6*. You will stimulate both lymph node areas twice. (See pages 196/230, 230, 233, 199 and 232.)

CHAPTER 11

AFTER A BODY-CUPPING TREATMENT

AFTER-CARE RECOMMENDATIONS

Products to Apply

I often recommend applying a favorite skincare or therapeutic product after cupping applications. There are many products that can provide a wonderful complement to this treatment for the body.

As with face cupping, the pores are open, and circulation is boosted, so anything applied at this time will be more effectively absorbed as the pores and circulation recede. However, although it is equally beneficial to cleanse the skin after body cupping, that may not be as accessible in many clinical settings. If you work in a spa with hydrotherapies available, then showering or cleansing the skin would be a nice after-treatment add-on before applying products. Alternatively, using warm towels to wipe the client down is an option, too. But if none of these cleansing options are available, don't worry, as it is not as necessary for the body-cupping treatment to receive similar absorption benefits.

There are also many great cellulite products on the market, as well as other therapeutic products to provide muscle relief or support the boosted circulation. You can find products with essential oils, herbal blends, or any high-quality product of choice in many stores, online or at wellness spa retail centers.

Another great option is choosing to apply body wraps or other mask-like products (such as cellulite masks) that will further enhance this cupping treatment. Or your client may prefer a more soothing product, like a seaweed mask, or perhaps a muscle-relaxing product such as arnica, after such a vigorous treatment. Whatever you recommend (or choose for yourself), be sure that nothing is too stimulating or continues the soft tissue manipulations for that day.

WHAT TO AVOID

As with face cupping, avoid excessive heat or cold applications as well as strong exfoliation or other aggressive skin treatments after body-cupping. See page 162 to review these suggestions.

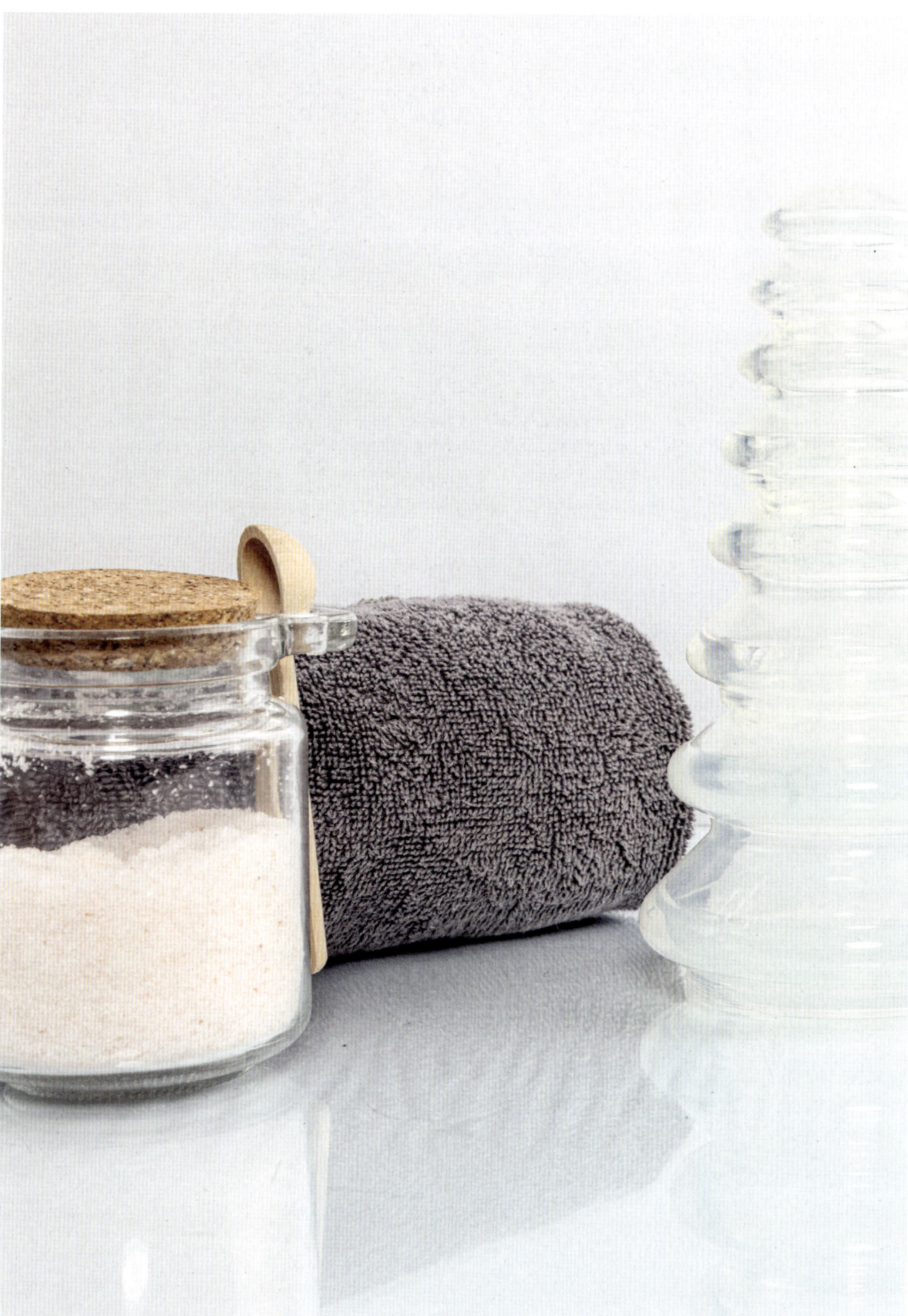

MAKE A TREATMENT PLAN

When cupping for cellulite reduction, less can truly be more with cups. Cellulite doesn't happen in a day, so it shouldn't be expected to disappear entirely in one treatment. Those who have used this modus operandi, and overworked the body either too long or too strongly to try to resolve cellulite as soon as possible, have subsequently seen bruising and swelling following a procedure. Yes, there will be positive results in the first session, but cumulative applications work best.

Cupping should not be done every day. Considering how disruptive cups can be to the preexisting state of anatomy, we must allow the body time to process what has been affected before applying cups again.

The skin has been stretched, pulled and manipulated by the cups. Allowing 48 hours is sufficient for the boost in circulation to settle, capillaries to relax and all the nutrients to settle into where they've been drawn (until the next time). Cupping daily can alter the skin's integrity, causing it to sag and stretch if overworked in this manner.

The circulation has been boosted and fluids are moving more efficiently after this cupping treatment. While this is extremely helpful, using cups too often can move too much fluid, ultimately causing swelling. The body should be allowed to process and settle for approximately 48 hours before reapplying cups.

The fascia, muscles and nerves have been manipulated and need time to process, too. While cups can yield great results, the area cupped may be sensitive to what has been treated. This is no different than deep-tissue therapies. How sensitive is the area the next day? Should it be worked again while in a state of discomfort? In these cases, the answer is no. It is strongly advised not to repeat an application in the same location within forty-eight hours.

Frequency

This treatment is intense for the entire body, even though at times it may not feel like it. Choose two days of the week separated by forty-eight hours, such as Monday and Thursday or Tuesday and Friday. The time between treatments is necessary for the tissue to fully process the work.

A treatment series is highly recommended for cellulite reduction. If possible, scheduling six to eight sessions within four to six weeks is a great treatment plan. Treatments twice a week for several weeks will show just how powerful these results can be when done in this cumulative manner. Take photos, measure areas of concern and observe the changes throughout the treatment process. The body will contour, surfaces will smooth and soft tissues will transform—all from the wonderfully therapeutic benefits that cupping offers!

Daily Consideration

If daily cellulite treatments are of interest, consider following the flow of lymph as instructed in this book with comforting massage strokes. Or perhaps try a simple dry skin brush treatment, which lightly stimulates the circulatory system and is great for daily use. Also, since manual lymph drainage is safe to experience on a daily basis, the option to receive MLD daily is always available.

FAQ

HOW LONG DO THE RESULTS LAST?

Every person will have a different outcome, and cupping results are most responsive when you follow all recommendations for application, timing and frequency. All cupping results are lasting, creating a permanent shift within the previously affected anatomy.

Yes, lifestyle choices play a role in the results and aging is inevitable. But if good choices are made for lifestyle improvement, and regular cupping bodywork is available, the potential for long-lasting, permanent results is available!

This treatment offers many great benefits for general wellness, and choosing to enjoy them can instill hope and enthusiasm for its true potential. Year after year, client after client, we see consistent results that confirm this is true. I hope this gets you excited to share the wonderful benefits of this amazing full-body-cupping treatment!

THE FULL POTENTIAL OF THERAPEUTIC CUPPING FOR SKIN HEALTH: MY STORY

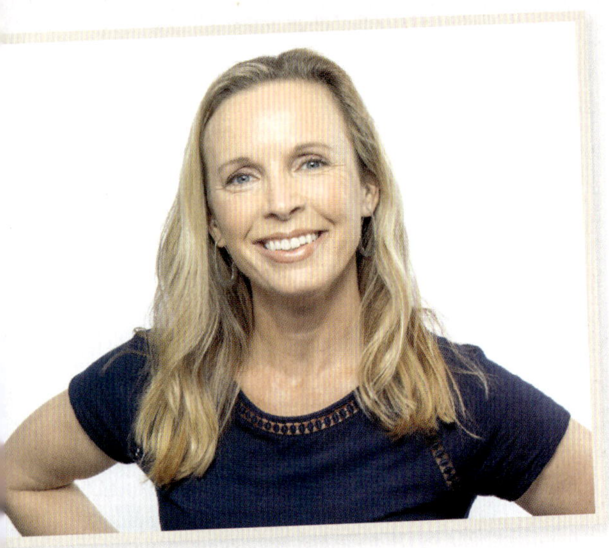

I have been a professional bodyworker since 1999. Therapeutic bodywork encompasses a number of techniques and modalities to promote health and wellness. In my case, cupping was one of the first alternative modalities I learned, and it completely changed everything for me, both personally and professionally.

In my clinical practice, cups have been the best addition to my therapeutic treatments. The way cups change soft tissue and the extraordinary results they bring my clients are unlike any other modality I have learned, ever. I have provided everything from relaxing treatments and deep-tissue bodywork to post-surgical rehabilitative therapies and even Thai massage. I am grateful to have a thriving practice that specializes in the fusion of cups with my existing professional skillset. Every client who receives cupping bodywork reports enjoyable sensations and incomparable results. The feedback I receive is always positive.

My personal story of cupping is what brought me to be the professional bodyworker and cupping instructor I am today.

At age eighteen, I suffered a major car accident that left me with many injuries, including a very large scar across the left side of my face. My face received dozens of stitches to repair it, and within the layers of healing skin remained bits of glass and sand from the impact. Much of my body suffered soft tissue damage also, leading to chronic pain patterns that Western medicine simply did not resolve.

While I was thankful to be alive, as a teenage girl, suffering from all the residual pains and knowing my face was disfigured were shocking, to say the least. The jaw pain and dysfunction that accompanied such an injury was just as traumatic.

I first experienced cups almost three years later. At that time, the body cupping tapped into points of pain and discomfort that other methods of therapy couldn't access, and the relief was immediate and extraordinary. And although it was an emotional experience for me to let someone touch my face with cups, the sensations and the visible results were quite dramatic in a positive, comforting way.

I began practicing cupping on a regular basis, following the muscle patterns and the natural lymph drainage pathways, learning what worked best for such treatments. Over many sessions, my hip, back and shoulder pain from the impact eased significantly. Additionally, my scars became less visible and the pain in my face diminished. Over time, some of the glass and sand that was stuck in my face came to the surface and was successfully removed.

My personal experience motivated me to become the cupping instructor I am. I have a strong desire to share this powerful information with as many people as I can. Every time I share my history, people have a hard time even identifying where my scar is until I point it out; cupping has helped heal my skin that much!

The face-cupping treatment I teach offers remarkable benefits to the skin on so many levels. It is truly one of the most amazing treatments I have ever received and shared. Because of this, I offer it in clinical settings for not only cosmetic enhancement, but for all the other health and functional benefits cupping offers. Face cupping is one of the most popular add-ons in my office. Whether it's for a general cosmetic boost, post-surgical recovery from cosmetic procedures, head traumas, sinus congestion, jaw tension or stress relief, once someone experiences it, they quickly proclaim how wonderful it is, not only for its cosmetic results but also as an experience within their skin unlike anything else. It really does feel that good!

Body cupping has offered incredible results for my personal clients, our students and their clients. Cellulite concerns resolve, gifting people with a renewed sense of confidence as well as pain relief associated with cellulite patterns. Similar applications of body cupping have initiated detoxification from medications, chemical afflictions and years of sluggish immune systems. This style of body cupping has also provided

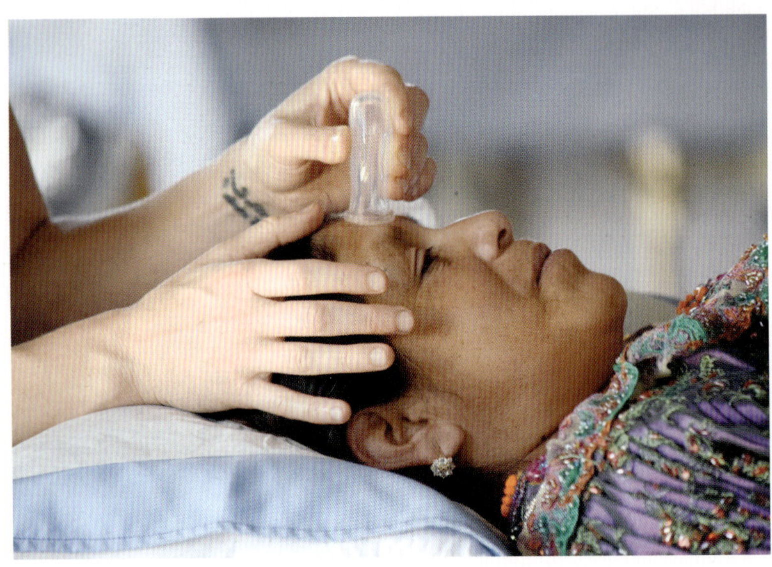

incomparable muscle relief to athletes and accelerated post-surgical recovery for patients. Time and time again, we have seen that such cupping treatments can bring about a wonderful new sense of health and well-being to those who have the chance to experience it.

On an even more personal level, I also do volunteer work in different countries, which has brought an entirely new appreciation for this cupping bodywork. In one volunteer program, we worked with orphaned girls in India who suffered all types of atrocities, both physically and emotionally. I remember meeting one dear girl who had many scars on her face. I showed her my scars, and her curiosity at my healed skin allowed me the chance to massage her face. Although I did not have my cups, a gentle massage following the lymph drainage pathways allowed her a chance to relax, and she welcomed some much-needed TLC to her face. At the next year's visit, I gave a copy of my first cupping book to the girls, and they had a great time flipping through the pages, seeing the photos and getting a look into what Aunty Shannon did for people. To this day, thanks to the internet, I am still in touch with a few of the girls and they enjoy seeing where I go and the work I do.

Another volunteer organization I work with serves underprivileged communities in Guatemala. This clinical outreach brings together acupuncturists, massage therapists and other alternative medicine practitioners, working together in a way unlike anything I have ever been a part of. People come seeking therapeutic relief from all sorts of burdens, from stress to physical abuse to severe injuries and sickness.

One year, a young boy came in with severe face trauma, a rare skin cancer on his face. At first, all that we could do for him was gentle lymph drainage. That first treatment got his circulatory systems moving, and the immediate results were reduced swelling and relaxation. At the next session, I worked more intently with him, using a combination of gentle hands and cups over his delicate face. The results were phenomenal. His skin health improved. The swelling in his face decreased so much that his once-obstructed eyes were now open and he could see. He smiled and played while we all fought tears of joy and accomplishment. That experience of working with him changed me forever as a face-cupping practitioner, as well as a human being.

From one of the most traumatic incidents of my life came a gift I am honored to share with the world. My hope with this book is to share the healing potential of therapeutic cupping for lymph drainage. I hope you too will discover not only the wonderful cosmetic benefits of these treatments but also how effective they are on a greater, therapeutic and holistic wellness level.

I wish you all the joy and gratification of sharing these cupping treatments and all the magic they truly offer, both for your clients and for you.

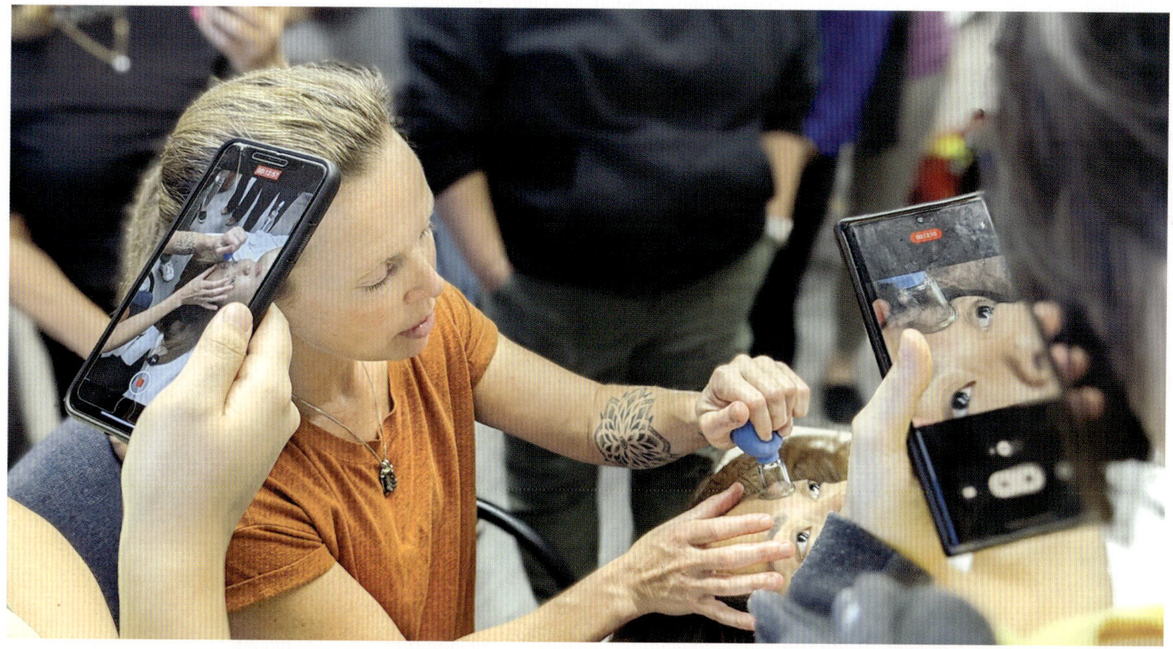

REFERENCES AND RESOURCES

ARTICLES

Al-Bedah, A.M.N., I.S. Elsubai, N.A. Qureshi, T.S. Aboushanab, G.I.M. Ali, A.T. Elolemy, A.A.H. Khalil, M.K.M. Khalil, and M.S. Alqaed. 2019. "The medical perspective of cupping therapy: Effects and mechanisms of action." *Journal of Traditional and Complementary Medicine* 9 (2):90–97. https://doi.org/10.1016/j.jtcme.2018.03.003

Mehta, P., and V. Dhapte. 2015. "Cupping therapy: A prudent remedy for a plethora of medical ailments." *Journal of Traditional and Complementary Medicine* 5 (3):127–34. https://doi.org/10.1016/j.jtcme.2014.11.036

Rozenfeld, E., and L. Kalichman. 2016. "New is the well-forgotten old: The use of dry cupping in musculoskeletal medicine." *Journal of Bodywork and Movement Therapies* 20 (1):73–8. https://doi.org/10.1016/j.jbmt.2015.11.009

Bentley, B. 2015. "A cupping mark is not a bruise." *The Lantern* 12 (2):14–20

Arslan, M., N. Kutlu, M. Tepe, N. Yilmaz, L. Ozdemir, and S. Dane. 2015. "Dry cupping therapy decreases cellulite in women: A pilot study." *Indian Journal of Traditional Knowledge* 14 (3):359–64

Moortgat P., M. Anthoniseen, J. Meirte, U. Van Daele, and K. Maertens. 2016. "The physical and physiological effects of vacuum massage on the different skin layers: A current status of the literature." *Burns & Trauma* 4:34. doi:10.1186/s41038-016-0053-9

HealthyHype.com. Retrieved October 2023. "Edema (swelling)and anasarca (generalized body swelling)." Post by Dr. Chris. http://www.healthhype.com/what-is-edema-body-swelling-pathophysiology-causes-types.html

Fogli, A. 1992. "Muscle orbiculaire et patte d'oie. Etude pathogénique et approche chirurgicale." ["Orbicularis oculi muscle and crow's feet: Pathogenesis and surgical approach."] *Annales de Chirurgie Plastique Esthétique* 37 (5):510–18

Prager, W. 2013. "Differential characteristics of incobotulinumtoxin A and its use in the management of glabellar frown lines." *Journal of Clinical Pharmacology* 5:39–52. doi:10.2147/CPAA.S37582

BOOKS

Amato, L., H. Bickmore, J. Doyle, M Nielsen, L. Sarfati, J. Schlaiss, and L. Todd. 2020. *Milady Standard Esthetics, 12th Edition.* Cengage Publishing

Wittlinger H., D. Wittlinger, A. Wittlinger, and M. Wittlinger. 2019. *Dr. Vodder's Manual Lymph Drainage: A Practical Guide, 2nd Edition.* Stuttgart: Thieme. doi:10.1055/b-006-161131

Földi, M., and R. Strössenreuther. 2005. *Foundations of Manual Lymph Drainage, 3rd Edition.* 2005. Elsevier Mosby Publishing

Black, A., and J. Hunt. 2017. *The Cellulite Myth: It's Not Fat, It's Fascia.* Post Hill Press

Gilmartin, S. 2017. *The Guide to Modern Cupping Therapy: Your Step-by-Step Source for Vacuum Therapy.* Robert Rose Publishing

RESOURCES

Opis Supplies: https://opis-supplies.ca (Canada only)

Carbo Medical Supplies: www.carbo.ca (Canada only)

Lhasa Oms: https://lhasaoms.com (USA only)

Modern Cupping Therapy Education Company: www.moderncuppingtherapy.com

ACKNOWLEGMENTS

Thank you to my loving family and friends for their continued support and patience with the process that is writing books.

To my mother, Jackie, for encouraging me every step of the way and knowing when a daughter just needs her mom sometimes. Love you, Mom.

To my father, Tom, for continuing to be the rock that is this girl's father, always reminding that all the struggles are totally worth it in the end. Love you, Dad.

To my brother, Jason, for always being there as a big brother and friend, urging me to just keep going. Love ya, Jay.

To my beautiful nephews Jacob and Evan for allowing me to be the aunty I love to be to some of my favorite humans. And to my other nephew, Ethan, always a loving star in my sky. Love you boys so very much.

And to dear Rafique, for your patience and support during these consuming writing times, and for sharing this adventure with me all the while. Love you, Rif.

To the Gilmartin and Leiby families I am honored to be a member of, and to all my friends for simply being there when and wherever I need you. In no particular order, special thanks to my lovely sister-in-law Paula Gilmartin, dear Marie Melia, Tanisha Balarezo, Mandy Pannone, Khadija Zahra, Susan Sandage, Dan "Jefe" Wunderlich and the Global Healthworks Foundation, Claudine Rousseau, Deena Taddia, Mark Pawley, Sasha Durandetto, Roger Perez, Kasandra Klein, Jacob Monn and Scott Cohen.

To Stacie Nevelus and Lauren Lane, for sharing in the educational adventures of MCT Education Company. And to all the students, clients, colleagues and cupping practitioners who help make this all possible—many thanks to you all!

To the Choong family and the Opis Acupuncture team, Carbo Medical Supplies and LhasaOMS for your continued product support.

To Doug Arcos for his excellence in photography, capturing all the beautiful images that created this book. Special thanks to Tammy Leiner with Longevity Centers of America for her support with thermographic imaging. And to Khadija, Kas, Eva, Dawn, Tanisha, Rif and Scott for your help with the photographs.

To Kathleen Fraser for her patient support as my editor, Kevin Cockburn and his team for their excellence in graphic design, the entire staff behind the scenes at Robert Rose who work to make the books come to life. And last but not least, to Mr. Bob Dees for believing in me from day one, and continuing to make me the author that I am today. Thanks for everything, Bob.

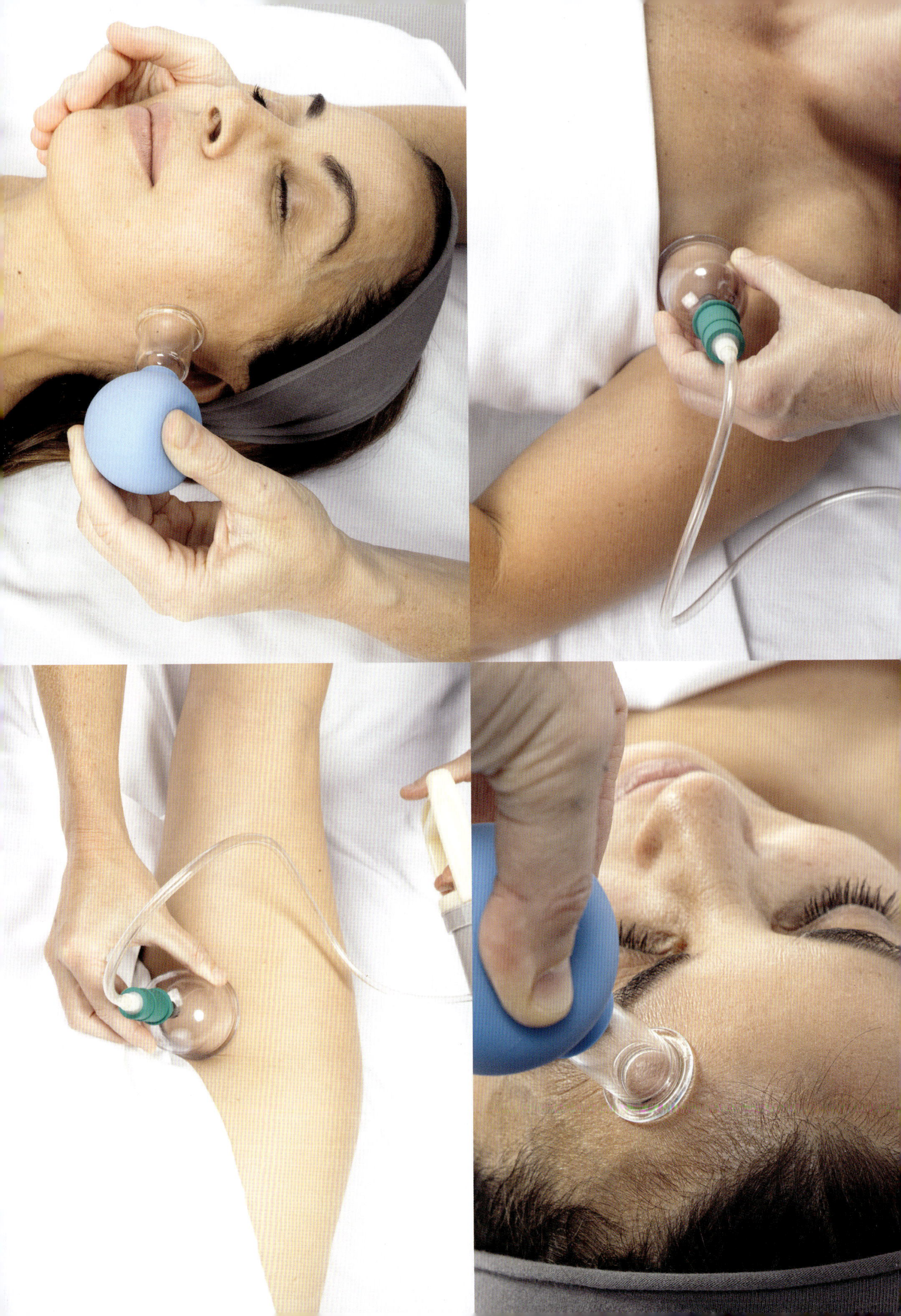

INDEX

Library and Archives Canada Cataloguing in Publication
Title: Face & body cupping : a step-by-step guide to lymph drainage for
professional cosmetic rejuvenation, cellulite reduction & contouring / Shannon
Gilmartin, CMT, CMLDT, CMCTPE.
Other titles: Face and body cupping
Names: Gilmartin, Shannon, author.
Description: Series statement: Modern cupping therapy series | Includes index.
Identifiers: Canadiana 20230545777 | ISBN 9780778807186 (softcover)
Subjects: LCSH: Cupping—Handbooks, manuals, etc. | LCSH: Face—Care and
hygiene—Handbooks, manuals, etc. | LCSH: Beauty, Personal. | LCGFT: Handbooks
and manuals.
Classification: LCC RM184 .G545 2024 | DDC 615.8/9—dc23